16.50

Cancer Care in the Community

Edited by Barry Hancock MD FRCP FRCR

YCRC Department of Clinical Oncology
Weston Park Hospital NHS Trust
Sheffield

with a Foreword by

Robert Grant
General practitioner
Markinch Medical C   e
Fife

PGMC 9/6/05

Radcliffe M
Oxford and

© 1996 Barry Hancock

Radcliffe Medical Press Ltd
18 Marcham Road, Abingdon, Oxon OX14 1AA, UK

Radcliffe Medical Press, Inc.
141 Fifth Avenue, New York, NY 10010, USA

British Library Cataloguing in Publication Data

A catalogue record for this book is available from the British Library.

ISBN 1 85775 0 934

Library of Congress Cataloging-in-Publication Data

Cancer care in the community/edited by Barry Hancock; with a
foreword by Robert Grant.
p. cm.
Includes bibliographical references and index.
ISBN 1-85775-093-4
1. Cancer—Patients—Care.   2. Community health services.
I. Hancock, Barry W.
RA645.C3C333 1996
362.1'96994—dc20
95-47756
CIP

Typeset by AMA Graphics Ltd, Preston
Printed and bound by
Biddles Ltd, Guildford and King's Lynn

Contents

List of contributors

S Ahmedzai	Professor of Palliative Medicine, Department of Surgical and Anaesthetic Sciences, University of Sheffield
B D Aird	Principal Consultant, KPMG, St James Square, Manchester (formerly Chief Executive, Weston Park Hospital, Sheffield)
R Akehurst	Professor of Health Economics and Director, Sheffield Centre for Health and Related Research, Sheffield
C Black	Research Sister, YCRC Department of Clinical Oncology, Weston Park Hospital, Sheffield
D Brooks	CRC (Cancer Research Campaign) Lecturer in Palliative Medicine, University of Sheffield, Royal Hallamshire Hospital, Sheffield
D Clark	Professor of Medical Sociology, Trent Palliative Care Centre, Sheffield
D Clegg	Information Manager, Trent Palliative Care Centre, Sheffield
R E Coleman	Senior Lecturer in Medical Oncology, YCRC Department of Clinical Oncology, Weston Park Hospital, Sheffield
A G O Crowther	Medical Director, St Luke's Hospice, Sheffield
S Dixon	Health Economist, Sheffield Centre for Health and Related Research, Sheffield
A Faulkner	Professor of Communication Studies, Trent Palliative Care Centre, Sheffield
B W Hancock	Professor of Clinical Oncology, YCRC Department of Clinical Oncology, Weston Park Hospital, Sheffield
M H Goyns	Senior Lecturer in Molecular Oncology, Institute for Cancer Studies, Sheffield
P C Lorigan	Lecturer in Medical Oncology, YCRC Department of Clinical Oncology, Weston Park Hospital, Sheffield
H Malson	Senior Research Fellow, Trent Palliative Care Centre, Sheffield
T W Noble	General Practitioner and Associate Specialist in Palliative Medicine, St Luke's Hospice, Little Common Lane, Sheffield
H C Orchard	Development Manager – Cancer Services, Weston Park Hospital, Sheffield

J Owen   Research Sister, YCRC Department of Clinical Oncology,
                  Weston Park Hospital, Sheffield
M H Robinson   Senior Lecturer in Clinical Oncology, YCRC Department
                  of Clinical Oncology, Weston Park Hospital, Sheffield

Foreword

No longer does medical input alone determine the quality of care obtained by the patient with cancer. In addition to the cancer specialist, physicians, surgeons and general practitioners; many nursing and paramedical specialists have major roles to play. Added to this hospital administrators and community health trust managers must ensure that their clinical departments are organized and re-sourced to deliver the highest possible standard of care, while the new wide spectrum of commissioning agencies must ensure that cancer services are purchased in sufficient volume to meet need, to agreed high quality standards and at tariffs that are affordable. Intermeshed with all of this are the widely varying but frequently crucial activities of a range of voluntary and charitable organizations providing input into research, care and treatment of cancer.

In this decade the drive to achieve optimum cure rates for various types of cancer has resulted in pressure to concentrate cancer treatment into regional centres of excellence, and there has at the same time been a desire to provide treatment as close to the patient's home as possible. Coinciding with the increasing success in the treatment of many cancers has been the introduction of major campaigns of cancer prevention and screening.

Cancer Care in the Community provides a comprehensive and concise review of all aspects of cancer management. In recognition that many of those involved in the management of hospitals, community health trusts and volun-tary organizations may come from non-medical backgrounds the accessibility of this text will allow them to obtain the essential background knowledge to make informed decisions regarding the future of their cancer services. The excellent sections in the text describing not only cancer treatment but also all aspects of supportive and shared care, including psychological aspects of the diagnosis and the influence of the diagnosis on other family members, are to be valued by all those involved in the day-to-day management of the cancer patient.

I recommend *Cancer Care in the Community* as an outstanding addition to the bibliography on cancer. From the MacMillan nurse to the cancer specialist, from the GP fundholder to the executives of major commissioning agencies, from the health council member to the directors of cancer charitable organiza-tions; all will find this book an invaluable reference in support of their work to improve the care and treatment of the cancer patient.

Robert Grant
October 1995

Acknowledgement

I would like to thank Sue Brown for all her help in the preparation of this manuscript for publication

List of abbreviations

αFP	alpha fetoprotein
ABVD	Adriamycin, bleomycin, vinblastine, dacarbazine
ADH	antidiuretic hormone
ALL	acute lymphoblastic leukaemia
AML	acute myeloid leukaemia
ATPase	adenosine triphosphatase
β-HCG	beta human chorionic gonadotrophin
CEA	carcinoembryonic antigen
CHART	continuous hyperfractionated accelerated radiotherapy
CHOP	cyclophosphamide, Hydroxydaunorubicin, Oncovin, prednisolone
CIN	cervical intraepithelial neoplasia
CMF	cyclophosphamide, methotrexate, fluorouracil
CNS	central nervous system
COIN	clinical oncology information network
CSF	cerebrospinal fluid
CRC	cancer research centre
CT	computerized tomography
DES	diethylstilboestrol
DGH	district general hospital
DHA	district health authority
DMSO	dimethyl sulfoxide
DNA	deoxyribonucleic acid
DSM	(diagnostic scale to determine depression)
ECG	electrocardiogram
FAB	French/American/British
FCE	finished consultant episode
FHSA	family health service authority
FIGO	Fédération Internationale de Gynécologie et d'Obstétrique

G-CSF	granulocyte colony-stimulating factor
GI	gastrointestinal
GP	general practitioner
HBV	hepatitis B virus
HIV	human immunodeficiency virus
HTLV	human T leukaemia/lymphoma
IACR	International Association of Cancer Registries
IARC	International Agency for Research on Cancer
LREC	local research ethics committee
MOPP	mustine, Oncovin, procarbazine, prednisolone
MRC	Medical Research Council
MRI	magnetic resonance imaging
NHS	National Health Service
NSAIDS	non-steroidal anti-inflammatory drugs
OPCS	Office of Population Censuses and Surveys
PCI	prophylactic cranial irradiation
PRN	pro re nata (as required)
PSA	prostate specific antigen
PTHrP	parathyroid hormone-related peptide
QALY	quality-adjusted life year
RCN	Royal College of Nursing
RHA	regional health authority
SCLC	small-cell lung cancer
SVC	superior vena cava
TENS	transcutaneous electrical nerve stimulation
TNM	tumour, node, metastasis
TPN	total parenteral nutrition
UV	ultraviolet
WHO	World Health Organization

The basic science of cancer

M H Goyns

What is a cancer cell?

Tumours and leukaemias consist of neoplastic cells, but the ways in which these cells differ from their non-malignant counterparts are not always clear. The most obvious difference is that cancer cells exhibit abnormal growth regulation, so that they appear to proliferate out of control. It is the gradual increase in numbers of malignant cells which eventually results in the emergence of a tumour or, in the case of bone marrow cells, in the appearance of a leukaemia. There are a number of features of the malignant phenotype, however, that are not obviously associated with increasing cell numbers, but which are equally important in allowing for the evolution of an aggressively metastasizing malignant cell population.

Recently it has become increasingly accepted that blocking the process of programmed cell death (apoptosis) is an important aspect of the malignant transformation of cells. It appears that all normal cells have the ability to undergo apoptosis and that this process has an important role to play in normal tissue development. In fact over 95% of all lymphocytes naturally undergo apoptosis as part of the normal function of the immune system. All cells have the ability to monitor damage to their DNA, and if such damage cannot be repaired then the cell appears to make a decision to enter apoptosis and to kill itself in a controlled manner. Cancer cells differ from normal cells in that they seem to have lost the ability to undergo apoptosis. Therefore damage to the DNA in malignant cells is not fully repaired and these damaged cells survive within a tissue with their mutations in place. If these mutations affect the proliferation control of the cell, then this immediately gives the malignant cell a growth advantage over normal cells.

All populations of cells in the body undergo differentiation, and cells in the epithelium and bone marrow do so on a regular basis. One of the underlying features of this process is that, as the cells become more differentiated, so their ability to grow and proliferate generally becomes reduced. It is therefore of interest that many malignant cells appear to be morphologically immature, as if they had been blocked at an early stage of differentiation, enabling them to continuously proliferate and build up in numbers.

Angiogenesis – the process of blood capillary formation – is restricted to areas of wound healing in the normal individual. However, tumour cells also have the ability to induce angiogenesis. This is a very necessary event if tumours are to grow aggressively as they need both a good supply of nutrients, oxygen and growth factors as well as an efficient way of removing damaging waste products.

Angiogenesis is also intimately related to what is perhaps the most important clinical aspect of cancer, namely metastasis. If cancer was simply characterized by the evolution of a single well defined tumour mass, then most cancers would be curable by surgery. It is the ability of cancer cells to spread through the body and to evolve into numerous secondary tumours in vital organs that makes this disease so difficult to treat. Cancer cells, unlike their normal counterparts, have the ability to travel to other tissues and to colonize them. This ability to metastasize is of course greatly aided if the cancer cells are able to induce angiogenesis, as new capillary growth into the tumour mass allows cancer cells access to the blood system.

The aggressively malignant cancer cell, therefore, exhibits several features which allow for its enhanced proliferation capacity and for its novel ability to spread to and colonize other tissues.

Cancer: a genetic disease

For many years it has generally been accepted that cancer is a gene-based disorder. There are now several lines of evidence that clearly support this idea and as such have led to a greatly increased understanding of how cancer arises and how it may be treated.

First, the vast majority of cancers appear to be monoclonal. This can be demonstrated by the presence in all malignant cells of a tumour of specific cell markers such as a polymorphic enzyme subtype or, in females, of an inactivated maternal or paternal X chromosome. The presence of such markers in all cancer cells from a particular tumour indicates that they have all arisen from a single ancestral cell.

Chromosomal changes are one of the most characteristic features of tumour cells and in some cases particular chromosome abnormalities are consistently associated with particular types of malignancy, for example the Philadelphia chromosome (which is one of the products of a reciprocal translocation involving chromosomes 9 and 22) with chronic myeloid leukaemia and translocations involving the chromosome 8q24 region with Burkitt lymphoma. These observations demonstrate that in cancer cells, genetic material can be gained, lost or rearranged.

Chemical carcinogens and radiation are mutagenic and their abilities as mutagens and carcinogens are closely linked. For example, 40 of the 4000 chemicals that have been identified in tobacco and tobacco smoke have been demonstrated to cause mutations in DNA and these are the same chemicals that have a tumorigenic effect. Damage to DNA therefore appears to be an essential event in the malignant transformation of cells.

There are a number of rare tumours that are associated with a clear inherited predisposition to malignancy. An example of this is retinoblastoma, which in its familial form occurs primarily in children. It should also be noted that there are other, more common, tumours which show a much weaker but nevertheless discernible familial predisposition, for example some types of colon, breast and ovarian cancer. Such conditions clearly imply that the information for a cell to become malignant is inherited and hence genetic.

The above observations have indicated that genes within normal cells may be altered as a prerequisite for the evolution of malignant disease. These genes have become known as oncogenes.

Oncogenes

An oncogene is an altered form of a normal gene, known as a proto-oncogene. The latter is a disparate grouping of genes, some related to one another, some completely unrelated, but all capable of being altered to form an oncogene. The protein product of a proto-oncogene has an important role in normal cell physiology. It is usually involved in regulating an aspect of cell growth, apoptosis and/or cell differentiation.

The oncogene is abnormal in that it produces too much or too little of its protein product, or it produces an abnormal protein. By convention each oncogene has usually been given a name based on a combination of three letters written in italics (e.g. *MYC*, *RAS*, *SRC*), although some closely related oncogenes are also distinguished from one another by an extra letter or number (e.g. *MYC*, *MYCL*, *MYCN*, *BCL-1*, *BCL-2*, *BCL-3*). Two general classes of oncogenes have been recognized. The first are the dominant-acting oncogenes (often simply called oncogenes), which require the alteration of only one of their two alleles within a cell for an oncogenic effect to occur. The second group are the recessive oncogenes (often called tumour-suppressor genes), which require that both of their alleles be deleted or mutated to allow for an oncogenic effect. Over 100 genes that can be classed as oncogenes or tumour-suppressor genes have now been identified.

Although oncogenes are essential for the evolution of human cancer, it is important to remember that a single oncogene will not cause cancer. Cancer is a multistage process and it is likely that an oncogene is necessary for each of these stages to occur. The involvement of more than one oncogene in tumorigenesis has been demonstrated by studies of colon carcinoma. It has been observed that the K-*RAS* oncogene occurs in a large proportion of these tumours and is usually mutated during the early stages of malignancy. Progress to full malignancy appears to depend on the mutation or deletion of the *P53* tumour-suppressor gene and metastatic ability on the loss of the *DCC* tumour-suppressor gene. There are likely to be other oncogenes that are also involved in this process. Some of the more common associations of oncogenes with human malignancies are shown in Table 1.1. Such studies are now allowing researchers to build up a framework of genetic changes that define the malignant evolution of a number of types of tumours and leukaemias.

Oncogene	Malignancy	Percentage of tumours containing altered oncogene
ABL (rearranged)	Chronic myeloid leukaemia	100
BCL-2 (rearranged)	Follicular lymphoma	45–80
ERB-B2 (amplified)	Breast carcinoma	30
K-*RAS* (mutated)	Colon carcinoma	50
MYC (rearranged)	Burkitt lymphoma	100
P53 (mutated or deleted)	Lung carcinoma	80–100
RB1 (mutated or deleted)	Retinoblastoma	100

Table 1.1:   Common associations of oncogenes with human malignant cells

Oncogenes and the malignant phenotype

An understanding of how the malignant cell phenotype may be defined in terms of oncogene involvement has been made possible by the discovery of the functions of the proteins coded for by the normal counterparts (proto-oncogenes) of the oncogenes and tumour-suppressor genes.

Oncoprotein	Function
SIS	Platelet-derived growth factor
HST	Fibroblast growth factor
ERB-B	Epidermal growth factor receptor
FMS	Colony-stimulating factor-1 receptor
KIT	Stem cell growth factor receptor
RAS	Membrane-associated ATPase
GSP	G_s protein
SRC	Membrane-associated protein tyrosine kinase
RAF	Cytoplasmic protein-serine kinase
ERB-A	Steroid receptor
FOS	Subunit of AP-1 transcription factor
JUN	Subunit of AP-1 transcription factor
MYC	DNA binding protein
P53	DNA binding protein

Table 1.2: Function of oncogene protein products

As the proto-oncogenes were isolated, and part or all of their nucleotide sequences determined, it proved possible to compare these sequences (and the amino acid sequences that they code for) with relevant computer data banks. This procedure has demonstrated that several of these protein products are identical to or have very close homology with known proteins. As a result it is now possible to identify which genetic changes are necessary for the emergence of different aspects of the cancer cell phenotype (Table 1.2).

As might be expected, uncontrolled proliferation of tumour cells is often associated with overproduction of growth factors or their receptors. It is therefore not surprising that several of the oncogenes code for such proteins. *SIS* codes for part of the platelet-derived growth factor, *ERB*-B for the epidermal growth factor receptor and *FMS* for colony-stimulating factor-1 receptor. The proliferation signal that is triggered by the action of a growth factor and its receptor is carried inside the cell by a series of proteins which eventually activate transcription factors (proteins that control the switching on or off of genes) in the cell nucleus. The *RAS* oncogene family has been shown to code for G-proteins that are typical of this intracellular signalling pathway and the oncogenes *JUN* and *FOS* code for subunits of the AP-1 transcription factor. In other words, all of these oncogenes (and many others beside), code for proteins that are involved in the regulation of cell growth and proliferation. These observations are very important as an alteration in the structure or level of any of these proteins could clearly contribute to uncontrolled proliferation.

The mechanism by which a cell enters apoptosis is not fully understood but a number of proteins have now been shown to be intimately involved in regulating this process. One of these proteins is coded for by the *BCL-2* oncogene which can be permanently switched on in lymphocytes as a result of a chromosome translocation. This has the effect of preventing the lymphocytes from entering apoptosis and thus increasing their cell life span, which in turn makes the lymphocytes more vulnerable to acquiring mutations in other oncogenes that regulate proliferation of these cells.

Blocks in the differentiation of cells also appear to be under the control of oncogenes. In acute promyelocytic leukaemia (M3) for example, a chromosomal translocation has been shown to alter the involvement of a glucocorticoid receptor in controlling the differentiation of these myeloid cells so that they are blocked at the promyelocyte stage of differentiation. This receptor is coded for by a member of the *ERB-A* oncogene family.

The induction of angiogenesis by tumour cells appears to be controlled by a number of growth factors but two that have been identified are the ligand for the *ERB-B2* receptor and a member of the fibroblast growth factor family (which is coded for by the *HST* oncogene).

Metastasis is a complex process which is probably mediated by a range of cell adhesion molecules and growth factor signalling systems. Several proteins have now been identified that are implicated in this process. Two of these have been identified and are coded for by tumour-suppressor genes. This means that both alleles of these genes are deleted or mutated and that functional protein is absent from the cell. In colon cancer it is the loss of the *DCC* tumour-suppressor gene that is associated with metastatic spread, whereas in melanoma the loss of the *NM23* gene appears to allow metastasis to occur.

Causes of cancer are mediated by oncogenes

It is now possible to gain an insight into how factors which are known to be important in the evolution of malignant disease have their effect. In all cases it has become increasingly apparent that the mechanisms underlying these events involve the activation of oncogenes or inactivation of tumour-suppressor genes.

A factor which appears to be frequently involved in tumorigenesis concerns inherited predisposition to malignancy. In rare cases this represents a strong predisposition with high penetrance and, in the case of children born into families affected by retinoblastoma, leads to a very high risk of their developing this cancer. It is now recognized that such individuals are at risk only if they inherit a deleted or mutated allele of the *RB1* tumour-suppressor gene, and any cell that subsequently loses or suffers a mutation in the other wild-type allele will gradually evolve into a tumour. Among the more common tumours, a number of predispositions of low penetrance have been identified. Recently these have been associated with mutations in a variety of genes that can be inherited, for example the *MSH2* gene in hereditary nonpolyposis colorectal cancer.

Diet has been implicated as a cause of cancer by many epidemiological studies that have been carried out in recent years. In some cases dietary components show a very strong link with cancer incidence. For example, aflatoxin (a fungal contaminant on certain foods) appears to be a major cause of liver cancer in some parts of the world and in this case has been closely linked to specific mutations in the *P53* tumour-suppressor gene in the malignant liver cells. A weaker though significant correlation has also been detected between high-fat/low-fibre diets and the incidence of colorectal cancer. In the latter case the molecular mechanisms are not so clear, but it is possible that such diets allow for a greater exposure of the cells of the large bowel to carcinogens in the diet, which in turn cause increased mutation rates in the oncogenes of these cells. It is clear that all colorectal tumours show mutations of *RAS* and /or *P53* genes.

There are well established links between smoking and a number of tumour types, particularly lung cancer. Several chemicals have now been identified in tobacco which will cause mutational damage to DNA and the presence of mutations in the K-*RAS* and *P53* genes in the majority of lung tumours more than suggests a causative link.

Radiation-associated carcinogenesis appears to be primarily a twentieth century phenomenon. Much of the information relating to this risk has been derived from studies of radiologists, uranium miners and survivors of the atomic bombs that were exploded in Japan. The recent dramatic increase in melanoma incidence has also implicated the ultraviolet component in sunlight. Although a great deal has still to be learned about the effects of radiation at the molecular level, some interesting correlations have been observed between radiation exposure and non-random chromosome abnormalities, which are a common mechanism leading to the activation of oncogenes.

Viruses are clearly important causative agents in a number of malignancies. The human papilloma virus has been demonstrated to inactivate the protein products of both the *P53* and *RB1* tumour-suppressor genes in cervical cancers. Hepatitis B virus is known to be important in the evolution of liver cancer and there is some evidence that it might integrate into the host cell genome near to the *ERB-A* oncogene and thus presumably disrupt the latter's activity. Epstein–Barr virus appears to play a causative role in the development of some lymphomas and interestingly one of its proteins has now been demonstrated to activate the *BCL-2* oncogene.

Clinical applications of oncogene research

Oncogene research has led to a much greater understanding of the nature of cancer and as a result has provided potential applications for the clinical management of cancer patients (Table 1.3). An important feature of this is the development of more effective counselling to prevent cancer. Prevention of cancer is clearly the favoured option when compared to the possibility of developing effective anti-cancer therapies. The identification of mutated forms of the *RB1* tumour-suppressor gene in families affected with retinoblastoma have already led to the establishment of counselling programmes for such family groups. Although this represents a small number of people, much work is currently under way to identify those oncogenes that have a weaker but much more widespread cancer-predisposing effect in the population. It is also now possible for the clinician or health worker to offer more authoritative advice on lifestyle options. The mechanism underlying tobacco-induced malignant disease is well established and the significance of dietary components in either increasing or reducing the risk of cancer is becoming better understood.

Once a patient presents with cancer, however, it is important to carry out an accurate diagnosis in order to gain useful information about prognosis. The oncogenes have now provided new possibilities for improving diagnosis. As the oncogenes are often rearranged forms of normal genes, they can be used as tumour-specific markers. For example, it has proved possible to use information about the rearranged *BCL*-2 oncogene in non-Hodgkin's lymphomas and *BCR–ABL* fused oncogenes in chronic myeloid leukaemia to develop very sensitive tests to detect minimal residual disease after treatment. Overproduc-

Oncogene abnormality	Clinical application
RB1 mutation or deletion	Counselling for risk of retinoblastoma in affected families
P53 mutation or deletion	Counselling for risk of lung cancer in smokers
P53 mutation	Early warning of colon cancer
ERB-B2 amplification	Marker of poor prognosis in breast cancer
BCL-2 rearrangement	Detection of minimal residual disease in lymphoma patients
BCR-ABL rearrangement	Detection of minimal residual disease in chronic myeloid leukaemia patients
ERB-A rearrangement	Development of DMSO-analogue therapy for acute pro-myelocytic leukaemia
ERB-B2 amplification	Development of antibody-based therapy for breast cancer

Table 1.3:   Potential clinical applications of oncogene research

tion of the *ERB-B2* oncoprotein in breast cancer cells has also been shown to be a reliable marker of poor prognosis and metastatic spread to the lymph nodes. One particularly interesting recent development has been the discovery that mutated *P53* genes can be detected in stool samples, which can alert the clinician to the early onset of colorectal cancer.

The development of novel anti-cancer therapies based on knowledge of the oncogenes has raised numerous exciting possibilities and our understanding of the structure – function relationships of oncoproteins may be used to devise a new generation of anti-cancer drugs. There are several chemicals that are currently being studied for their activity in blocking growth factor stimulation of cells and for specifically interfering with the activity of the mutated but not the normal *RAS* proteins. As several oncoproteins are associated with the cell membrane and have extracellular domains, it is possible that monoclonal antibodies raised against such proteins could be used specifically to attack the malignant cells. This approach has already had some clinical success by using anti-*ERB-B2* antibodies in combination with *cis*-platinum to treat breast cancer.

There appear to be many encouraging lines of investigation based on oncogene research and, taken together, these hold out the promise of future innovative improvements to the clinical management of cancer patients.

Summary

- Cancer cells show uncontrolled proliferation for several reasons, including altered growth control, blocks in apoptosis, differentiation arrest, angiogenesis and metastasis.

- Cancer is a gene-based disorder and is mediated by the activity of oncogenes and tumour-suppressor genes.

- The protein products of the oncogenes and tumour-suppressor genes are involved in all aspects of the malignant phenotype.

- Knowledge of oncogenes and tumour-suppressor genes is now being used to develop useful diagnostic aids and in the future may lead to new anti-cancer therapies.

Further reading

Franks L M and Teich N M (1991) *Introduction to the Cellular and Molecular Biology of Cancer*, 2nd edn. Oxford University Press, Oxford.

2

Cancer facts and figures

D Clegg

Introduction

The prevalence of cancer, its diagnosis, treatment and final outcome, has been the subject of increasing public awareness and interest throughout the twentieth century. In tandem with this has been a growing commitment to cancer prevention as well as to cure and palliation. This has been demonstrated particularly within the developed world.

After coronary heart disease, cancer is the most common form of death. About one person in three in England and Wales will develop cancer at some stage in their life; approximately one person in four will die as a result. In 1988 there were around 300 000 newly diagnosed cases registered within the UK. In 1992 nearly 165 000 people died from cancer.[1]

It has been stated that the treatment of cancer accounts for about 7% of all NHS expenditure, amounting to about £1000 million per year at 1986/87 prices.[2]

Developments in the planning of health care provision, and growing emphasis on financial management, have given increased focus to the study of trends of cancer incidence and mortality and to the active promotion of cancer prevention. This was given a high priority in 1985 with the development of the Europe Against Cancer Programme. This aims at reducing the numbers of deaths from cancer by 15% by the year 2000. The UK's *Health of the Nation* document also aimed at disease prevention and health promotion, with cancer forming one of the five target areas.[3]

This chapter discusses trends in cancer incidence and mortality worldwide, with particular emphasis on the UK. The role of the cancer registries is reviewed, especially in the light of growing demand for reliable information in the planning of services and in audit. Finally, known risk factors are summarized, together with a brief overview of preventative measures currently in use or under investigation.

Cancer registration

The importance of epidemiology in cancer research has been widely recognized for many years, with mortality figures available for at least a century. However, there has been much discussion on the relative value of considering trends in mortality or trends in cancer incidence when assessing progress against cancer.[4,5] Mortality statistics reflect the impact of cancer on patients who die of the disease, but do not record the experience of those patients who survive. Falls in mortality may reflect a decreased incidence of the disease and/or improved survival through earlier diagnosis or improved treatment. Declines in cancer rates may indicate reduced exposure to risk factors. However, they may also reflect increased detection and treatment of pre-cancerous conditions through improved screening programmes.

The collection of data on diagnosis of cancers was initiated at a number of sites worldwide earlier this century, especially during the 1930s. Since that time an increasing number of countries have embarked on the collection of cancer morbidity data. Improvements in the quality and detail of information have been observed which are reflected in the expansion and coverage of the series of volumes *Cancer Incidence in Five Continents* promoted by the International Agency for Research on Cancer (IARC) and the International Association of Cancer Registries (IACR).[4] The growing use of computers in cancer registration is marked, and this has led to improvements and innovation with direct entry of data from a variety of sources.

The first system in England and Wales to collect statistics about cancer incidence and mortality commenced in 1929. It monitored the outcomes of cancer patients treated with the then new radium therapy. Of prime importance was the use of statistical information in the planning of services. Complete national coverage was achieved in 1962.

There are 11 independent regional registries located within England, and the Welsh Office is responsible for the registration of all patients within Wales. There is a similar system of registration within Scotland, based on five regional registries. It is anticipated that there will be some amalgamation of registries within England to reflect the recent NHS reorganization. However, it should be remembered that the *Review of the National Cancer Registration System* recommended that the position of the cancer registries be safeguarded and cancer registration be maintained as a core activity if regional responsibilities were to be changed. The regional registries regularly submit notification of registered patients to the Office of Population Censuses and Surveys (OPCS).

Items of information for collection are formed into a 'minimum data set' which has substantial overlap with the NHS's minimum data set. Nonetheless, items may be specified which can prove difficult to collect in practice and completeness may vary with region. Information may be obtained from local hospitals (medical records, pathology reports and others identified by registry staff), FHSAs, GPs on request, the private sector and various screening programmes, and by referring to death certificates. Additional information is recorded through active and passive follow-up.

In 1990, the *Review of the National Cancer Registration System* highlighted the value of the system and made recommendations to promote improvements, especially in the light of the need to plan for and evaluate the implementation of new treatments and screening procedures and to estimate cost-effectiveness.[6] Among other things it recommended developing links between cancer registry data and other NHS databases; establishing automated links with computerized pathology reports; and linking specialized tumour registries and lists of patients enrolled in trials with the regional and national system. Emphasis was also given to the development of a core standard data set for the national system as noted above.

Notwithstanding the role of the cancer registries in the UK, there is continuing demand for high-quality data collection on patients with cancer. One of the driving forces behind this is the need to detect early errors made in the administration of radiotherapy and/or chemotherapy through a programme of quality assurance and audit. There is much debate on the best way to achieve this. Pollock (1994) noted that many 'stand alone' systems developed for clinical audit do not allow for comparisons between clinicians, across districts or providers. Furthermore, they often fail to allow for linkage with cancer registries or other routine data systems.[7] These systems lack a population focus and are not standardized. A more sophisticated approach is taken in the proposed Clinical Oncology Information Network (COIN). This would focus on clinical information comprising details of diagnosis, investigation and treatment of all patients referred to cancer treatment centres within Britain. It is intended to support audit and to give early warning of hazardous practices. Fundamental to COIN is the development of clinical core data sets for oncology, coordinating clinical guidelines and standard setting. COIN's proponents maintain that there is no existing structure available to realize these key aims.[8] However, the proposal for a new information system has not met with universal acclaim. Basnett *et al.* (1994) argued that such a system would depend as much as Korner and the cancer registries on returns of clinical data and that errors in such data result from poor case notes.[9] They go on to recommend the improvement of current systems including the cancer registries, rather than the duplication of them.

Pollock advocated encouraging clinical audit systems capable of complementing a population focus and integration with the cancer registries and routine hospital data systems.[7]

Against this background, developments nevertheless continue. A new programme is under way within the West Midlands RHA based on the existing data collection networks in the cancer registry and cancer centres, with additional links between the CRC Trials Unit and the registry.[10] It is intended that the resources of the cancer registry be used to maximum advantage whilst being of value to clinicians in their local practice.

Demography

The United Kingdom

In the UK, cancer is the second highest cause of death after coronary heart disease. In 1990 it accounted for some 25.4% of deaths.[11] The incidence of most types of malignant neoplasms increases with age and cancer is seen particularly as a disease of the elderly. More than 70% of all new cases occur in the over-60s.[1] The death rates for male and female tend to be broadly similar though there are differences with age. Mortality figures for 1988 (Figure 2.1) show a higher number of female deaths in the band 25–54 years. This reflects the relationship between age and some types of malignancy, in this case the incidence of cancer of the breast and cervix. From the age of 55 to 84, the male death rate outstrips the female.

Cancer is also one of the most common causes of death in children aged 1–14, with leukaemia having the highest death rate, followed by malignant neoplasm of the brain.[6] Nevertheless, it should be remembered that new treatments have reduced the number of deaths in children by more than half over the last two decades.[11]

The highest incidence of any type of cancer continues to be lung cancer, with nearly 44 000 cases diagnosed within the UK in 1988. Some 39 000 people died of the disease in 1992 – nearly a quarter of all cancer deaths. More men than women die from the disease. The highest overall cause of mortality amongst women is breast cancer. However, there are regional variations, with more women dying from lung cancer in parts of northern England and Scotland.[1] The incidence of the most common forms of cancer is shown in Figure 2.2.

Trends in overall cancer mortality in England and Wales during the last 30 years show little overall improvement. Mortality has increased in the elderly population but has declined in younger age groups. There has been a noticeable

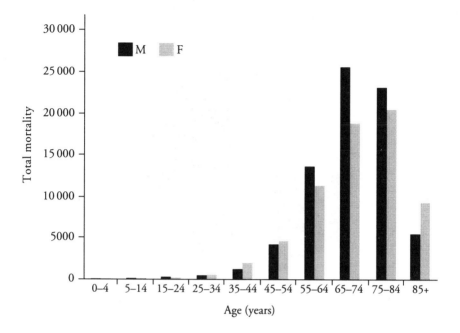

Figure 2.1: Mortality from malignant neoplasms in England and Wales in 1988.

decline in death from stomach cancer during the period, but death from lung cancer has shown a complex pattern. With the exception of the very elderly (80–84 years), deaths in men are declining. This pattern is repeated for younger women. However, for women over the age of 60 there is a growing death rate from lung cancer.[12]

In her excellent series of papers, Austoker[12] also pointed to the increasing incidence of a variety of other cancers. Some of these may be due to improved diagnosis and increased life expectancy. However, a genuine increase may be observed for prostatic cancer, which was the third greatest cancer diagnosis in men after lung cancer and non-melanoma skin cancers in 1988. It resulted in the second highest number of cancer deaths for men in 1992. As can be seen in Figure 2.3, incidence is rare prior to the age of 45 but then increases rapidly. An increase in incidence is also seen for testicular cancer, which is the commonest cancer among young men. Incidence figures for 1988 in England and Wales show a peak around the 25–29 year age group (Figure 2.4). Increased incidence is also seen for cervical cancer in young women and in melanoma.

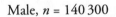

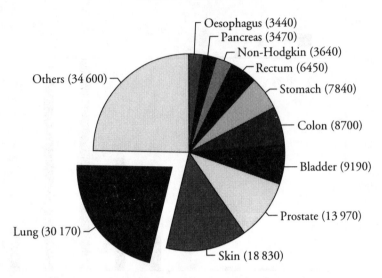

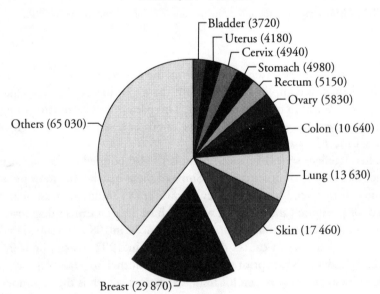

Figure 2.2:   New cases of cancer in the UK in 1988 (adapted from Austoker, 1994).

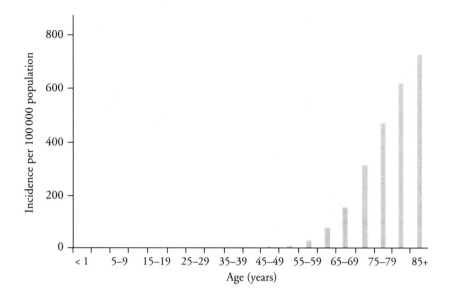

Figure 2.3: Incidence of prostate cancer in England and Wales in 1988.

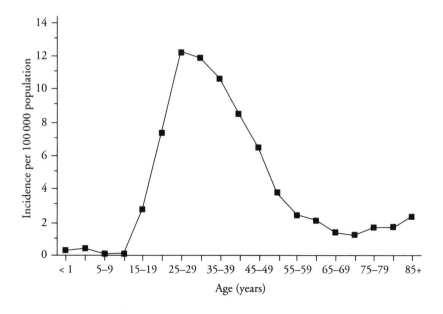

Figure 2.4: Incidence of cancer of the testis in England and Wales in 1988.

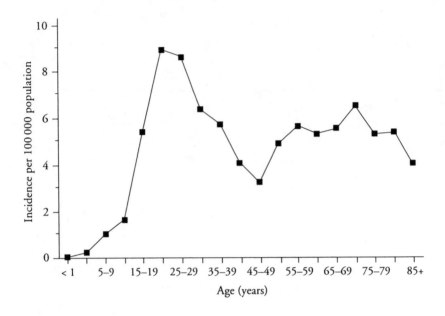

Figure 2.5:   Incidence of Hodgkin's lymphoma in England and Wales in 1988.

A number of cancers show a bimodal incidence by age. Typical among these is Hodgkin's disease, with peaks in the 20s and the early 70s (Figure 2.5).

It is notable that incidence rates in certain epithelial cancers are higher in men than in women.[2] Figures for England and Wales in 1988 (Figure 2.2) show a higher incidence of cancer of the lung, stomach, rectum, oesophagus and bladder. Incidences for cancer of the gallbladder and pancreas were broadly similar between males and females and a slightly higher rate of cancer of the colon in females was observed. Nearly three times as many females were diagnosed with cancer of the thyroid during the period.

It has not proved possible to examine the impact of ethnicity on cancer incidence within the UK to date. However, with the inclusion of data on ethnic origin within the 1991 census, analysis should prove possible in the future.

The international context

Trends in cancer incidence and mortality within England and Wales show certain parallels with other developed countries. On the other hand, there are marked differences when comparing certain cancers with the Far East and some

Eastern European countries. These differences are due largely to varying risk factors between populations, and the sophistication or otherwise of screening and cancer control programmes.

In their review of overall cancer incidence, Higginson *et al.* reported that stomach cancer was the most important cancer for both sexes combined in 1980.[20] It is now estimated to be the second most common after lung cancer.

Incidence of lung cancer is continuing to increase worldwide, being the most common in Europe, North America, Australia and countries of the former Soviet Union. Japan, the Caribbean and South America also have high incidence. Coleman *et al.*, when considering trends within Europe, noted increasing incidence in Poland, Hungary, former Czechoslovakia, Romania and former Yugoslavia in comparison with other more northern and westerly European countries.[5] This is mirrored with increases in cancers of the oral cavity, pharynx and oesophagus, which are all cause for concern. Increasing risk of these cancers is also seen in Germany and Denmark. Some decrease in risk has been observed in Finland. In developing countries, the picture varies with level of cigarette smoking. In 1980, lung cancer did not appear in the top five cancers prevalent in Western Africa. However, there are increases observed for men in Singapore, Hong Kong, Kuwait and Brazil, where smoking is increasing.[13]

As has already been noted, there is a decline in stomach cancer in England and Wales. This is reflected worldwide, with the possible exception of China. Nevertheless, it is still the most frequent cancer in Japan. High rates are also reported in Korea and other Eastern Asian countries, China, the former USSR and parts of Latin America.

Colorectal cancer is seen as a disease of economically developed countries. Whilst incidence is increasing slightly in Northern and Western Europe and in North America, mortality figures are generally decreasing. This contrasts with the picture in Eastern Europe and Asia, where both are generally increasing.[5]

In contrast, the preponderance of liver cancer is seen in developing countries, with high incidence in sub-Saharan Africa, East and South-East Asia and Melanesia. There is low incidence in South America, Australia and New Zealand (except in Maoris and Polynesians).[13]

The incidence of cancer of the mouth and pharynx is high in Southern Asia, being the first in men and third in women in 1980. They are very common in Indian populations and have been associated with the chewing of betel nuts.

Incidence of oesophageal cancer varies widely around the world, with high risk in Northern Iran, Turkestan, Kazakhstan, Uzbekistan, Western and Northern China, South Eastern Africa and parts of South America. Large decreases in incidence have been seen in Singapore, Shanghai and Hong Kong in recent years.[5]

Breast cancer is the most common cancer in women. However, incidence varies considerably. High risk areas include North America and Western Europe, whilst women in Japan and China have much lower risk.[13] Cervical cancer is the second most common female cancer but is noticeably more prevalent in developing countries, where it is the leading female cancer.

Trends in cancer incidence and mortality are a complex area and it must be remembered that there is a wide range of influences, some of which will be considered in this chapter. Those wanting a more comprehensive discussion of worldwide trends in cancer are referred to *Trends in Cancer Incidence and Mortality*.[5]

Risk factors

The causes of cancer are numerous and interrelated and may be broadly classed as either environmental or genetic. 'Environmental' is used here to cover a wide range of influences, including chemical, occupational, social and biological factors. To complicate matters the cause of many cancers may be multifactoral in origin. The aim of this section is to give a broad summary of the major influences in cancer aetiology.

Environmental factors

Tobacco use is one of the major social factors in the development of cancers worldwide and offers a major target area for cancer prevention. It is implicated in cancers of the lung, upper respiratory tract, upper digestive tract, pancreas, bladder and renal pelvis and is suspected as a risk factor in the aetiology of cancer of the cervix, stomach and in some leukaemias.[13,14] It is estimated that around 30% of cancer deaths are attributable to tobacco use and reduction of smoking forms a major target of the UK's *Health of the Nation* policy.[3] Duration of smoking is a critical factor. The risk of developing cancer is reduced through stopping smoking and decreases substantially after five years. Smokers of pipes and cigars appear to have a lower risk of developing lung cancer than cigarette smokers. Exposure to low levels of tobacco smoke may also increase risk. There is a higher risk of cancer from the use of black tobacco found in Mediterranean and Latin American countries over blond tobacco.[15] Smoking *bidis* is a higher risk factor for cancer of the oral cavity than smoking cigarettes. Chewing tobacco and the use of small packets of snuff held between the cheek and gum also increases risk of oral cancer.[13]

Alcohol use is another major cause of cancer and it is estimated that around 3% of cancer deaths in the UK are related to excessive alcohol consumption, with as much as 10% in some countries.[16] Alcohol consumption increases the risk of developing cancers of the oral cavity, pharynx, larynx, oesophagus and liver. There is conflicting evidence over the role of alcohol consumption in cancers of the stomach, rectum and colon. There is some evidence that heavy drinking may increase the risk of breast cancer. Alcohol consumption has also been shown to act synergistically with smoking in all the sites noted above except for cancer of the liver, where the evidence is less consistent. Heavy smokers who also drink heavily have been shown to have a high cancer risk.

The level of impact of diet on the development of cancers is the subject of much investigation and results to date are not conclusive. However, evidence does indicate that diet may play a part in the development of cancer of the stomach and large bowel. It may also be implicated in breast and prostate cancer.[17] Most notable is the evidence for the protective effect of a high intake of fruit and vegetables. This protection is believed to reduce risk for cancer of the oral cavity, lung, oesophagus, stomach, colon, rectum, bladder and cervix. No protective effect is seen with hormonal cancers. Evidence for the protective effect of an increased fibre intake against colorectal cancer is confused, with no protective effect seen from cereals but some evidence of protection from vegetable fibre. High fat intake has been implicated in an increased risk for colorectal cancer and there is some evidence that the risk of prostate cancer may also be increased. Implications of high fat intake on breast cancer remain to be resolved, but it is established that obesity is a risk factor for endometrial and postmenopausal breast cancers.

A correlation between the presence of naturally occurring aflatoxins produced by fungal strains in contaminated food and the incidence of liver cancer has been seen, as has high level exposure to ochratoxin in Balkan nephropathy.[18] Conversely, there is no evidence to link food additives, such as preservatives, flavourings, colourings or artificial sweeteners, with cancer development.[17]

Socio-economic status is a significant determinant of risk in the development of cancer. Studies in the UK have shown that working-class groups have a higher risk of developing most cancers. It has been reported that this can be as much as 40% higher in unskilled manual workers (social class V) than in professional groups (social class I). This is more marked for men than for women. Increased incidence and mortality is particularly marked for stomach, lung, larynx, liver, oesophagus and oral cancers in men of lower socio-economic status. Men in higher social classes have higher incidence of malignant melanoma, cancer of the testis and of the brain, and Hodgkin's disease. Women from lower socio-economic groupings are more susceptible to cancer of the cervix, oesophagus, stomach, larynx and lung. However, certain cancers are much more prevalent in higher socio-economic groupings, breast cancer, for example, with almost 50% higher incidence in the highest social class than the lowest. Differing reproductive patterns between these groups seem to play a part in this effect. Women in higher socio-economic groups also experience higher levels of malignant melanoma, ovarian cancer and Hodgkin's disease.[19] Occupation type and unemployment are also determinants of risk, together with differences in lifestyle such as smoking and alcohol use, and dietary and sexual habits noted elsewhere. Religious teaching also affects lifestyle, which in some cases affect cancer risk. The low level of penile and cervical cancer in Jews, for example, is ascribed to circumcision. Reviews of the literature also indicate poorer survival in lower socio-economic groupings.

Changes in susceptibility to certain cancers can be associated with sexual behaviour and reproductive habits. Early experience of intercourse and number of sexual partners have been reported to increase risk of cervical cancer, which may reflect increased exposure to a sexually transmitted agent (see the section on viral agents, p. 24.) Recent studies indicate that, as well as female sexual behaviour influencing risk, male sexual history may be a determinant in their partner's susceptibility to cervical cancer.[20] Recent studies have also indicated that there is an increased risk with increasing number of pregnancies.

On the other hand, studies also suggest that increasing number of pregnancies has a protective affect against cancer of the breast, ovary and endometrium. Early first parity is also shown to have a protective effect against breast cancer in some studies, whilst births after 35 are believed to increase risk. Women experiencing late menopause have an increased risk of breast and endometrial cancer. Early menarche may also increase risk of breast cancer. Long-term breast-feeding appears to exert a protective effect against breast cancer.[20]

A number of naturally occurring and synthesized chemicals have shown causal links with cancer development. Exposure may be through a variety of sources such as occupational hazards, air and water pollution, food and drink, and via drug therapy. Examples of these agents are shown in Table 2.1.

There are many examples of 'occupational cancers'. Often they have been shown to be multifactoral in origin, whilst others can be traced to a single agent. Over 200 years ago a link between exposure to coal soot in chimney sweeps and their high incidence of scrotal cancer was noted by Percival Pott. Earlier this century links between increased incidence of cancers of the skin, bladder and respiratory tract and the coal gasification and coke production industries were suggested and later confirmed. All of these are multifactoral in origin. A notable single environmental agent is asbestos. First suspected as injurious to health in

Agent	Cancer site	Occupation
Alkylating agents		
Cyclophosphamide	Bladder	
Melphalan	Marrow	
Aromatic amines		
4-Aminodiphenyl	Bladder	Dye manufacturers, rubber
benzidine	Bladder	workers, coal gas
2-Naphthylamine	Bladder	manufacturers
Arsenic	Skin, lung	Copper and cobalt smelters, arsenical pesticide manufacturers, some gold miners
Asbestos	Lung, pleura, peritoneum	Asbestos miners, textile manufacture, insulation, shipyard workers, gas fitters, plumbers, carpenters and electricians (from Peto *et al.*, 1995)
Benzene	Marrow	Workers with glues and varnishes
Bis (chloromethyl) ether	Lung	Makers of ion exchange resins
Busulphan	Marrow	
Cadmium	Prostate	Cadmium workers
Chromium	Lung	Manufacturers of chromates from chrome ore, pigment manufacturers
Chlornaphazine	Bladder	
Immunosuppressive drugs	Reticuloendothelial system	
Ionizing radiations	Marrow and probably all other sites	Radiologists, radiographers
	Lung	Uranium and some other miners
	Bone	Luminizers
Isopropyl alcohol	Nasal sinuses	Isopropyl alcohol manufacture
Mustard gas	Larynx, lung	Poison gas manufacturers
Nickel	Nasal sinuses, lung	Nickel refiners
Oestrogens		
Unopposed	Endometrium	
Transplacental (DES)	Vagina	
Parasites		
Schistosoma haematobium	Bladder	
Chlonorchis sinensis	Liver (choangioma)	
Phenacetin	Kidney (pelvis)	
Polycylic hydrocarbons	Skin, scrotum, lung	Coal gas manufacturers, roofers, asphalters, aluminium refiners, those exposed to certain tars and oils
Steroids		
Anabolic (oxymetholone)	Liver	
Contraceptives	Liver (hamartoma)	
UV light	Skin, lip	Farmers, seamen
Vinyl chloride	Liver (angiosarcoma)	PVC manufacturers

Table 2.1: Chemicals linked with cancer (adapted from Doll and Peto, 1981)

the late 1800s, the need to reduce exposure in mining and manufacture was widely accepted by the 1930s. Nonetheless, the impact of low-level exposure was not widely appreciated until after World War II. Asbestos is known to increase the risk of lung cancer and mesothelioma of the pleura and peritoneum. Incidence of, and mortality from, mesothelioma was previously expected to show a levelling off and then a down-turn due to preventative strategies. However, recent work reported by Peto *et al.* indicates that mesothelioma deaths in the UK will rise for at least 15 years and more likely 25 years.[21] This is due to a continuing increase in the death rate in men under the age of 50 who began work in the 1960s, alongside the continuation of the trends already noted for men starting work in the early 1950s. Peto predicts that the eventual scale of the mesothelioma epidemic in the UK will outstrip that of the USA, which has already reached its peak.

Ultraviolet (UV) radiation has been implicated in the incidence of skin cancers. There is increasing incidence and mortality from malignant melanoma in fair-skinned populations which has been partially attributed to exposure to UV radiation. Adjustments in intensity and frequency due to changes in the ozone layer have been put forward as a possible increasing risk factor for skin cancer in the future.[15] The UK is targeting a reduction of ill health and death due to skin cancer in its *Health of the Nation* document. Ionizing radiation has been shown to give rise to a number of cancers. Exposure to radiation from nuclear weapons, either from blast or fallout, diagnostic and therapeutic procedures (especially prior to the 1960s) and through occupation (such as to radon in mining and in the nuclear industry) have all been implicated. Studies investigating the effects of electromagnetic fields indicate an increased incidence of cancers, especially leukaemia, in those who have been exposed through occupation.[26] Studies of residential exposure have shown less consistent findings.

A number of viral agents have also been associated with cancer. They may act by directly transforming a normal cell into a malignant one; in this case presence of the virus is required for the cancer to develop. In other cases, the virus is only required in the early phase of cell transformation and may considerably predate the development of disease. Table 2.2 gives a summary of viral agents and the diseases with which they may be linked.

Genetic factors

Genetic factors also play a major role in carcinogenesis, either alone or acting together in varying degrees with environmental factors. In hereditary diseases, such as Wilms' tumour and bilateral retinoblastoma, the presence or absence of

Virus	Cancer
Hepatitis B (HBV)	Hepatocellular carcinoma
Herpes simplex virus type 2	Possible link to cervical cancer
Human papilloma virus	Cervical cancer
	Benign warts
Epstein–Barr virus	Burkitt's lymphoma
	B-cell lymphomas
	Undifferentiated and poorly differentiated nasopharyngeal carcinoma
Human T-lymphotrophic virus type 1 HTLV-1	Adult T-cell leukaemia lymphoma
Human T-lymphotrophic virus type 2 HTLV-2	Hairy cell leukaemia
HTLV-5	Cutaneous T-cell leukaemia
HIV-1	Kaposi's sarcoma
Cytomegalovirus	Kaposi's sarcoma

Table 2.2:   Viral agents linked with cancer (adapted from Macdonald and Ford, 1991)

a specific gene may give a high (80–90%) chance of developing cancer. In another group of preneoplastic syndromes, somewhere in the region of 10% of people with the genetic malfunction may develop malignant disorder.[15] Detailed consideration of the molecular aetiology of cancer is given in Chapter 1.

Cancer prevention and screening programmes

The reduction of cancer incidence and mortality is one of the major targets of health promotion campaigns in the developed world in recent years. Governments, companies, communities, primary health care teams and individuals all have a role to play. Improved management of risk factors and hence reduction in incidence may be obtained via enhanced education programmes (primary prevention). Improved survival rates are assisted by early detection of existing conditions or cancer precursors and prompt intervention (secondary prevention). The European Community focused on this theme with their 'Ten commandments' in the European Code Against Cancer (Table 2.3) It has been suggested that, if respected, this code could lead to a decrease of about 15% in cancer incidence in the EU by the year 2000.

1   Do not smoke. Smokers, stop as quickly as possible and do not smoke in the presence of others.
2   Moderate your consumption of alcoholic drinks – beers, wines and spirits.
3   Avoid excessive exposure to the sun.
4   Follow health and safety instructions at work concerning production, handling or use of any substance which may cause cancer.
5   Frequently eat fresh fruit and vegetables, and cereals with a high fibre content.
6   Avoid becoming overweight, and limit your intake of fatty foods.
7   See a doctor if you notice a lump or observe a change in a mole, or experience abnormal bleeding.
8   See a doctor if you have persistent problems, such as a persistent cough, a persistent hoarseness, a change in bowel habits or an unexplained weight loss.
9   Have a cervical smear regularly.
10 Check your breasts regularly, and if possible undergo mammography at regular intervals above the age of 50.

Table 2.3:   European Code against Cancer (the 'Ten commandments')

A   To reduce the death rate for breast cancer in the population invited for screening by at least 25% by the year 2000 (from 95.1 per 100 000 population in 1990 to no more than 71.3 per 100 000).
B   To reduce the incidence of invasive cervical cancer by at least 20% by the year 2000 (from 15 per 100 000 population in 1986 to no more than 12 per 100 000).
C   To halt the year-on-year increase in the incidence of skin cancer by 2005.
D   To reduce the death rate for lung cancer by at least 30% in men under 75 and 15% in women under 75 by 2010 (from 60 per 100 000 for men and 24.1 per 100 000 for women in 1990 to no more than 42 and 20.5, respectively).

Table 2.4:   *'Health of the Nation'* targets (breast, cervix, skin and lung cancer)

In the UK, targets have been set to reduce ill health and death caused by four cancers: breast, cervix, skin and lung (Table 2.4). In addition, targets set for coronary heart disease which focus on alcohol consumption and diet may also affect on cancer incidence.

Education

Education of the public in risky aspects of their lifestyle forms a major plank of health promotion. There is, however, a notable gap in the UK government's existing policy, since a ban on tobacco advertising does not form part of the strategy to achieve the *Health of the Nation* targets.

The role of primary care teams is important to the success of *Health of the Nation*. Brief interventions lasting 5–10 minutes have proved to be effective for smoking and alcohol use in at least some patients. These interventions include assessment of level of use, brief advice specific to each person to stop or reduce use, and provision of written information and self-help books. Nicotine replacement may be offered to aid giving up smoking. The adoption of an action plan may be considered, with target dates set for reduction or cessation. This may be supplemented by a written contract between doctor and patient, especially when trying to stop smoking. Follow-up appointments to discuss and assess progress may also be offered. Practitioners may find varying reactions from patients, from welcoming to resentful. Successful interventions for smoking may be only 1 in 20, whilst brief advice on drinking may lead to a reduction of 25–35%. Hence the role of advice giver and supporter may not be seen as very rewarding and opportunities to give advice may be under-utilized. With the current level of knowledge on the impact of diet on cancer incidence, advice on diet needs to be individually tailored. It may be supplemented with leaflets on basic dietary issues.[14,16,17]

Development of a strategy for improved public awareness of the risk of ultraviolet radiation in the development of skin cancer is an aim of *Health of the Nation*.

Screening

Several screening programmes are in use or under investigation for a number of cancers. In order to be considered effective, procedures must be seen to reduce mortality and to be cost-effective, both to the health services and to the individual being tested. The benefits and disadvantages have been summarized (see Table 2.5).[22]

Screening for cancer of the cervix has proved effective in a number of countries, with notable declines in incidence and mortality being seen after programmes were introduced. The benefit has been summarized as a 75% decrease in incidence over 15 years in most countries where widespread screening has been implemented.[5] Sharp falls in incidence and mortality were seen in Iceland, Finland, Sweden and parts of Denmark after screening was introduced.[23]

Screening, if carried out correctly, can greatly reduce the risk to individual women. However, it has been reported that women at higher risk due to lifestyle or socio-economic status are less likely to attend for screening.[13] To be effective,

Benefits
- improved prognosis for some cases detected by screening
- less radical treatment for some early cases
- reassurance for those with negative test results.

Disadvantages
- longer morbidity in cases where prognosis is unaltered
- overtreatment of questionable abnormalities
- false reassurance for those with false negative results
- anxiety and sometimes morbidity for those with false positive results
- unnecessary medical intervention in those with false positive results
- hazard of screening tests
- resource costs: diversion of scarce resources to screening programme.

Table 2.5:   Benefits and disadvantages of screening[23]

programmes need to set up and maintain follow-up, referral and treatment systems, which may be met best by central organization. Screening was first introduced in the UK in the 1960s, with computerized call and recall systems being introduced in 1988. It is open to women aged between 20 and 64 years, with recall at least every five years. Women over 65 whose previous two smears were not negative are also recalled. Combined development of good practice and encouraging women to be screened are priorities of *Health of the Nation*.

Screening for breast cancer also underpins one of the main aims of *Health of the Nation*. Mammography has been proved to be effective in the reduction of mortality in individuals allocated to screening in randomized controlled trials. Evidence to support this is significant in women aged 50 and over, with a combined estimate from all randomized trials showing an overall reduction in mortality of 28%.[24] For younger women the position is less clear, with no reduction in mortality noted after five years in some studies; longer-term benefits remain to be seen. There is very slight risk from exposure to radiation in the procedure which is dependent on the dosage and age at screening. In the UK, women aged 50–64 are invited for screening every three years, with women over 65 being screened every three years on request. Again, reduction in breast cancer death in the screened population is targeted in *Health of the Nation*.

Self-examination for breast cancer has been widely encouraged through the European Code and elsewhere. However, the evidence for its efficacy in reducing mortality has yet to be fully established. As a result of this, Austoker recommends that until this is proven, its use as a primary screening technique should not be promoted.[24] Nonetheless, some studies suggest that those women who find smaller breast cancers have a better prognosis and there is a case for women to be more 'breast aware'.

Three tests for diagnosing colorectal cancer have been investigated. Digital rectal examination is simple but of limited value since a high proportion of tumours are outside the range of an examining finger. Faecal occult blood tests are under trial in Denmark, Sweden and the UK. They are cheap and easy to perform. However, research to date indicates that they have a low sensitivity and are only moderately acceptable to patients. In the light of the evidence to date, it is unlikely that faecal occult blood tests will be considered to form part of a screening programme in the UK until ongoing studies report their findings.[25] Notwithstanding this, screening by digital examination and faecal occult blood tests has been public policy in Germany since the 1970s.[5] Flexible sigmoidoscopy allows for the detection of benign adenomas which may in time become malignant, and thus this may be a more effective method of prevention. It is sensitive to small lesions and these may often be amenable to removal at the time of screening. Evidence accumulated thus far suggests that this method may prove an effective screening test and further trials are proposed to investigate its potential further. It is widely used as a screening procedure in the USA.

Screening for stomach cancer using air contrast photofluorography has been widely used in Japan since the 1960s. Some shift towards diagnosis of the disease at an earlier stage has been noted and those patients with cancers detected through screening appear to have better survival rates.[5] However, no controlled trials have been undertaken to substantiate the success of the Japanese programme.

A variety of screening procedures have been investigated for ovarian cancer. Two which show promise are a combination of prescreening with serum Ca 125 and selective ultrasound, and secondly transvaginal ultrasonography. A multi-centre trial on the second has just begun.[22]

Several tests have also been used to detect prostate cancer but have not provided clear evidence of efficacy. There is also concern over the ethics of screening for the disease, with more potential harm than benefit for patients with preclinical diagnoses that are unlikely to progress. The psychological consequences of this and for those with false positive diagnoses may be significant. In addition, screening may potentially lead to only a few additional years of life.[22]

Screening techniques have also been investigated for a variety of other sites, including bladder, liver, skin (melanoma), oral cavity and endometrium. The potential for these has yet to be established.

References

1   Austoker J (1994) Cancer prevention: setting the scene. *BMJ*. **308**: 1415–20.

2   UKACR (1994) *Cancer Registry Handbook*. UK Association of Cancer Registries, London.

3   Department of Health (1992) *Health of the Nation*. CM1986. HMSO, London.

4   Waterhouse J A H (1992) Introduction. In *Cancer Incidence in Five Continents, Vol 6* (eds D M Parkin, C S Muir, S L Whelan *et al.*), IARC Scientific Publications 120, IARC, Lyon.

5   Coleman M P, Esteve J, Damiecki P *et al.* (1993) *Trends in Cancer Incidence and Mortality*. IARC Scientific Publications 121, IARC, Lyon.

6   OPCS (1990) *A Review of the National Cancer Registration System. Series MB1 no. 17*, HMSO, London.

7   Pollock A (1994) The future of cancer registries. *BMJ*. **309**: 821–2.

8   Karp S J (1994) Clinical Oncology Information Network. *BMJ*. **308**: 147–8.

9   Basnett I, Pollock A and Gill M (1994) Collecting data on cancer. *BMJ*. **308**: 791.

10 James N and Lawrence G (1994) Future of cancer registries. *BMJ*. **309**: 1514.

11 MRC (undated) *Cancer*. MRC, London.

12 Austoker J (1994) Current trends and some prospects for the future – 1. *BMJ*. **309**: 449–52.

13 Tomatis L (ed.) (1990) *Cancer: Causes, Occurrence and Control*. IARC Scientific Publications 100, IARC, Lyon.

14 Austoker J (1994) Smoking and cancer: smoking cessation. *BMJ*. **308**: 1478–82.

15 Bosch FX (1990) Etiology. In *Manual of Clinical Oncology* (eds D K Hossfeld, C D Sherman, R R Love *et al.*), UICC, Geneva.

16 Austoker J (1994) Reducing alcohol intake. *BMJ*. **30**: 1549–52.

17   Austoker J (1994) Diet and cancer. *BMJ*. **308**: 1610–14.

18   Higginson J (1993) Environmental carcinogenesis. *Canc* (Suppl.). **72**: 971–7.

19   Kogevinas M (1992) Social inequalities and cancers. In *Preventing Cancers* (eds T Heller, L Bailey and S Pattison), Open University Press, Milton Keynes.

20   Higginson J, Muir C S and Munoz N (eds) (1992) *Human Cancer: Epidemiology and Environmental Causes*. Cambridge University Press, Cambridge.

21   Peto J, Hodgson J T, Matthews F *et al*. (1995) Continuing increase in mesothelioma mortality in Britain. *Lancet*. **345**: 535–9.

22   Austoker J (1994) Screening for ovarian, prostatic, and testicular cancers. *BMJ*. **309**: 315–20.

23   Austoker J (1994) Screening for cervical cancer. *BMJ*. **309**: 241–8.

24   Austoker J (1994) Screening and self examination for breast cancer. *BMJ*. **309**: 168–74.

25   Austoker J (1994) Screening for colorectal cancer. *BMJ*. **309**: 382–6.

26   Cardis E (1992) Ionising radiation. In *Human Cancer: Epidemiology and Environmental Causes* (eds J Higginson, C S Muir and N Munoz), Cambridge University Press, Cambridge.

Further reading

Doll R and Peto R (1981) *The Causes of Cancer*. Oxford University Press, Oxford.

Macdonald F and Ford C H J (1991) *Oncogenes and Tumour Supressor Genes*. Bios Scientific, Oxford.

3

Education, screening, prevention and surveillance

B W Hancock and P C Lorigan

Introduction

It has been estimated that one-third of cancers are preventable and one-third curable if diagnosed and treated early. It is therefore appropriate to reiterate the importance of education, screening and prevention (see also Chapter 2).

Education

Fear is a significant cause of delay in patients with cancer seeking medical attention. This fear is easily understood as many people still regard all forms of cancer as incurable. It is crucial to stress that many forms of cancer are curable if they can be detected at an early stage and that cure rates for early cancers are being further improved by the use of extra (adjuvant) treatment at the time of diagnosis. Adjuvant treatment in common cancers such as breast and colorectal carcinoma could save a significant number of lives each year.

Apart from fear, there are a number of other reasons why patients with cancer may present with advanced rather than early disease. Ignorance, misconceptions and embarrassment are significant factors in this category. Patients may mistakenly believe that a lump is only important if it is painful, or that an 'ulcer' is due to poor hygiene. The mass media play an increasingly important role in educating the general public about cancer, but tend to rely on general and dogmatic statements. Other forms of education, for example via women's groups, can usefully target at-risk groups of individuals and give good personalized service, but cannot hope to reach the numbers of people reached by the mass media. It is obvious that all these forms of education have their part to play if we wish to improve the general public's appreciation of the need to pick up and act on symptoms and signs of cancer at an early stage. From a purely financial point of view, education programmes are expensive, but failure to pick up cancer at an early stage results in major expenditure on the treatment of advanced disease and loss of earning capacity by the patient. Vast sums of money are spent on research and management of advanced disease; perhaps we ought to look more into preventive measures, since after all prevention is better than cure.

Prevention

It is now well established that a number of agents are carcinogenic. Chapter 1 dealt with known occupational carcinogens. However, the case is a lot less clear for a number of dietary and environmental factors. An association between viruses and malignancy was first noticed at the beginning of the twentieth century (Table 3.1). Only a limited number of these actually cause cancer in humans and only a few patients affected with these viruses go on to develop cancer (HIV excepted); other factors are almost certainly involved. For certain viruses, viral DNA either encodes for or activates a host oncogene. For others the mechanism for malignant change could be multitudinous. Again the best way to approach this problem is to prevent it and vaccines to Epstein–Barr virus and hepatitis B have been developed.

Direct physiological manipulation is being attempted in some malignancies; for example, young women who are at high risk of breast cancer due to strong family history may benefit from prophylactic tamoxifen. This is the subject of a large randomized study at present. Gene therapy may have a role in

Virus	Cancer
Hepatitis B	Hepatocellular carcinoma
Human papilloma virus	Cervical cancer
Epstein–Barr virus	Burkitt's lymphoma
	Nasopharangeal carcinoma
	Post-transplant lymphoma
HIV	Kaposi's sarcoma
	Non-Hodgkin's lymphoma
HTLV-1	Adult T-cell leukaemia/lymphoma

Table 3.1:   Viruses associated with cancer

the prevention of hereditary cancers, but this would involve germ line manipulation and many people consider this unethical. Despite all the expensive new techniques which may have a role to play, we are still finding it difficult to bring about the cheapest and most effective methods of prevention, such as encouraging people to stop smoking.

Screening

The basic principle of screening healthy people for cancer is that tumours are detected at an earlier stage when the tumour load is lower and therefore easier to eradicate (Table 3.2). This is a premise which is well founded on basic principles of cancer treatment. The major benefits of screening are that more people are cured of the disease than would otherwise be, and that this cure is achieved using less radical and less costly treatment. In addition, those who are found to be 'all clear' are reassured. There are, however, disadvantages to screening. Patients with 'borderline' abnormalities which would normally have regressed may be overtreated, there are problems with false-positive and false-negative test results, and patients are labelled as having a disease for a lot longer since it is caught earlier in its natural history. In addition, the costs of screening must be taken into account. Screening tests must satisfy a number of criteria: they must be sensitive (i.e. pick up the vast majority of people who have the disease) and specific (only test positive when the disease is present). Ideally the test should be validated in randomized studies and it should be cheap and simple to carry out, easy to interpret and reproducible. There must be the facility to act upon positive results promptly and a well designed course of action for borderline results. The ideal frequency of screening must be determined and the general population must be educated and made aware of the availability.

Screening for breast cancer is now established throughout the UK for women in the 50–65 age range in whom bilateral mammography is recom-

	Early	Late
Breast	75%	< 10%
Colorectal	90%	< 30%
Bladder	70%	< 30%
Cervix	> 75%	5%
Larynx	90%	20%

Table 3.2: Prognosis (five-year survival) in early and late cancer

mended every three years. The introduction of routine breast screening has led to the development of dedicated screening clinics with radiological, surgical and pathological input for rapid diagnosis. Screening has led to an increase in the detection of small tumours, in situ lesions and those of special histological type. It is now established that when screening mammography is performed as recommended, and with high-quality techniques, the mortality from breast cancer can be reduced by about 30% in those invited for screening. With 15 000 deaths due to breast cancer each year, this translates into a significant number of lives saved. Trials of screening mammography in young high-risk patients are in progress.

Invasive squamous carcinoma of the uterine cervix is generally preceded by in situ malignant change for ten years or more and because of this routine cervical smear examination has been introduced to screen for the disease. Although only about one-third of cases with in situ changes progress to malignancy, cervical screening can detect those at high risk, so treatment or close follow-up can be instituted. Dysplastic and in situ changes are generally treated by either colposcopy or cone biopsy of the cervix. Routine cervical smear testing has been associated with marked decline in the incidence and severity of invasive cervical carcinoma; in Britain the incidence has fallen by about 30%.

It is recommended that all sexually active women below the age of 50 have a cervical smear at 3–5 year intervals. Unfortunately women at particularly high risk often have the poorest compliance for screening programmes.

Attempts have been made to screen for other common cancers. For example, because ovarian cancer presents so late, attempts have been made to screen for this tumour using serum CA125 measurements and abdominal or trans-vaginal ultrasound scans. Unfortunately, apart from perhaps those with a strong family history, routine screening cannot yet be justified.

Our understanding of the molecular basis of cancer is increasing rapidly. We will soon have identified and cloned a number of genes implicated in many familial cancers. Over and above this, a number of genes (oncogenes and tumour-suppressor genes) which are contributory factors in the development of cancer have been identified. It is fair to assume that our ability to screen for the potential to develop cancer will increase greatly over the next ten years. The practical, moral and ethical issues which this will raise will be considerable. For example, the genes responsible for a number of familial cancers have been identified. These vary in penetrance: those with low penetrance are not associated with a high risk of developing cancer, but may be very common in the population and so contribute to the overall cancer load. Penetrance itself may depend on a number of genetic and environmental factors. The *BRCA1* gene accounts for about 5% of all cases of breast cancer. Women with the *BRCA1* mutation have an 85% lifetime risk of breast cancer and also an increased risk of ovarian cancer. The *BRCA1* gene is located on chromosome 17 and has been cloned. A routine test for the *BRCA1* gene is not yet available but should allow us to identify women at risk and offer advice on screening and treatment.

The following cancers have been identified as having chromosomal associations:

- familial breast/ovarian cancer – chromosome 17

- retinoblastoma – chromosome 13

- familial polyposis coli – chromosome 5

- hereditary non-polyposis coli – chromosome 2

- familial malignant melanoma – chromosome 9.

Surveillance

In assessing the need for follow-up surveillance in patients after treatment, three factors are important:

- knowledge of the biology of the tumour

- the pros and cons of follow-up for the patient and doctor

- the importance of teamwork.

The behaviour of many malignancies is now understood and is predictable – they may be potentially curable (e.g. children's tumours, lymphoma, uterine cancer), usually incurable (e.g. brain, lung) or have a very long natural history (e.g. breast, ovary).

In favour of follow-up is the fact that the patient and clinician will get the psychological reassurance that all is well, and the patient will be seen at an early stage of any recurrence of the disease. Proper follow-ups also allow accurate statistics. Long-term follow-up is particularly important for children, adolescents and young adults treated for curable cancer, since the incidence of late side-effects is increasing and there is a need to monitor these patients for these problems (e.g. growth or endocrine defects, chronic organ toxicities, second cancers). Against follow-up is the possibility that patients may be anxious or uneasy about continuous follow-up, that cured patients will be followed unnecessarily, that follow-up is time-consuming, and that even if things go wrong the clinician cannot always correct them.

The value of the community health service in follow-up cannot be over-emphasized. GPs, nurses and social workers all have an important role, particularly when they work in close liaison with the hospital oncology service. It is now usually accepted as important for shared follow-up to occur, perhaps initiated or led by a senior hospital oncologist but in close communication with other hospital specialists and with the GP and community health team. The oncologist or GP knows the patient well and will be able to detect slight but significant changes when the patient is seen and relevant history-taking and examination can be undertaken. Malignant disease is now accepted as the great mimic and any symptom or sign should be taken as relevant to the primary cancer or its treatment until proven otherwise. Psychological aspects of follow-up are all important; some patients will be followed unnecessarily and others may be well for periods from weeks to decades after therapy. Patients may not seek medical advice spontaneously but when abnormalities are found at follow-up there is a good chance that something positive can be done, possibly with further curative treatment, if not with palliative measures.

Further reading

Austoker J (1994) Cancer prevention: setting the scene. *BMJ*. **308**: 1415–20.

Austoker J (1994) Current trends and some prospects for the future – 1. *BMJ*. **309**: 449–52.

Austoker J (1994) Smoking and cancer: smoking cessation. *BMJ*. **308**: 1478–82.

Austoker J (1994) Reducing alcohol intake. *BMJ*. **308**: 1549–52.

Austoker J (1994) Diet and cancer. *BMJ*. **308**: 1610–4.

Austoker J (1994) Screening for ovarian, prostatic and testicular cancers. *BMJ*. **309**: 315–20.

Austoker J (1994) Screening for cervical cancer. *BMJ*. **309**: 241–8.

4

Treatment of cancer

M H Robinson and R E Coleman

Radical or palliative treatment

In the treatment of malignant disease, it is important to determine in each individual case whether cure of the disease is possible or probable. If cure is likely, the inevitable side effects and local reactions to treatment are more than justifiable. On the other hand, if cure is unlikely, it is vital that treatment offers improvement in the symptoms present, without the addition or substitution of significant symptoms from the treatment itself, and the probable side effects and local reactions to treatment must be carefully weighed against the expected benefits. This applies equally well to all forms of cancer therapy. The choice of the appropriate treatment is determined by the specialist(s) working with the patient and their support team. They use their understanding of the disease process and available treatments to select the programme which maximizes the patient's quality of life.

Surgery

The first therapeutic attempt is always the best (and sometimes the only) opportunity for cure of malignant disease. It is of the utmost importance, therefore, that the initial treatment is carefully considered. The known or likely extent of the disease, its expected response to the forms of treatment available, and its expected long-term behaviour all warrant assessment.

Surgery is the oldest method of treating malignant disease, but only in the last century has it become safe and effective with the greater appreciation of anatomical and physiological principles, the development of aseptic rather than antiseptic procedures, and the use of greatly improved anaesthetic agents and techniques.

Choice of treatment

It may be that surgery, either alone or combined with radiotherapy and/or cytotoxic chemotherapy, offers the best chance of eradicating the disease. For some malignancies, particularly those in the 'radioresistant' group, surgery is usually the only form of radical treatment available; though with the development of new cytotoxic agents and regimens, these are becoming more important in the overall management of the disease.

Radical surgery

Radical surgery may result in little deformity or dysfunction, or alternatively significant physical and functional impairment may ensue. All surgical procedures carry some risk of operative morbidity and mortality, and in situations where a choice of treatments is available these must be carefully assessed. The general physical and medical state of the patient is also highly relevant to the form of management selected.

Tumour resection en bloc may offer the best opportunity for cure, where this is feasible without unacceptable morbidity or mortality. It may include removal of the regional lymphatic glands (block dissection) if these contain demonstrable deposits or there is a high risk of involvement.

Other treatments in radical surgery

Some radical surgery procedures, e.g. radical mastectomy for early breast cancer, have been demonstrated to be unnecessary in the majority of patients. Its use was based on the theory that breast cancer was a loco-regional disease rather than a systemic one. In many women it has been supplanted by wide local excision and the use of postoperative radiotherapy. Simple mastectomy is another alternative.

Radical surgery for carcinoma of the uterine cervix was established by Wertheim. This operation involves removal of the uterus, a cuff of vagina, the fallopian tubes and ovaries, the broad ligaments and the pelvic lymph glands and lymphatics. This cannot be achieved entirely en bloc because of the need to carefully dissect out and preserve the ureters.

Abdominoperineal resection of the rectum for adenocarcinoma is also well established as a radical procedure. The involved section of bowel, with a generous margin proximally, and the associated mesentery and lymph glands are removed up to the level of the inferior mesenteric artery. Partial colectomy with removal of the mesentery and the lymph glands draining the affected segment likewise is a standard operation for colonic cancer.

For operable gastric carcinoma total gastrectomy, again with removal of the draining lymph glands, is undertaken. In selected cases of thyroid cancer, total thyroidectomy is appropriate. For operable involved lymph glands in one side of the neck from an ipsilateral primary tumour in the head and neck, radical neck dissection of the lymph glands, lymphatic channels, internal jugular vein and sternomastoid muscle offers a chance of cure.

Adjuvant surgery

In situations where surgery alone is not potentially curative, it may nevertheless play a useful part in the management of the disease. Planned removal of a large primary tumour as a preliminary to radiotherapy and/or cytotoxic chemotherapy may be of great benefit by reducing the bulk of tumour to be treated. Clear examples of this are seen in head and neck cancer, where advanced lesions of the laryngopharynx require radical surgery which alone has a very small probability of curing the patient. Adjuvant radiotherapy is often used to eradicate residual microscopic disease in this situation.

Palliative surgery

Surgery may be of great value as palliation alone. A colostomy for lower large-bowel obstruction from an advanced tumour may result in immediate relief of distressing symptoms. A tracheostomy for laryngeal obstruction may avert rapid death from asphyxia. A bypass operation for internal hydrocephalus caused by cerebral tumour may provide rapid relief of severe headaches, nausea and vomiting.

Diagnostic surgery

Diagnostic surgery may be of help in obtaining tumour tissue for histological diagnosis. This may take the form of a simple operation such as an excision of a lymph node or a more major procedure.

Radiotherapy

Radiotherapy is second only to surgery in importance as a treatment for cancer. Approximately 45% of patients with cancer will receive radiotherapy at some time during their illness. Radiotherapy is used either alone or in combination with surgery or chemotherapy.

Basis of radiotherapy

The origins of radiotherapy date back to the 1890s, when Becquerel discovered natural radioactivity and Roentgen discovered X-rays. Following Becquerel's discovery the Curies extracted a radiation-emitting element from pitchblende – radium. Radiation causes ionization in both normal and malignant tissue which damages the DNA causing subsequent cell death. Radiotherapy damages both normal and malignant cells, but the therapeutic advantage is achieved because more damage is inflicted on tumour cells than normal cells by a given dose of radiation, and because normal tissue is more able to recover following treatment. The use of fractionated radiotherapy (giving a total dose in small daily doses) improves the therapeutic ratio further. The impact of radiotherapy on a given tumour mass depends on a combination of its radiosensitivity, the potential proliferation rate and the cell loss factor. Radiotherapy planning involves the use of multiple radiation fields to deliver the prescribed dose to a defined volume containing the tumour and regions of potential spread whilst minimizing the dose to surrounding normal tissues.

Types of therapy

The forms of radiation currently available to the radiotherapist, and well established in practice, are shown in Table 4.1.

Radiotherapy is usually given in the forms of X-rays, gamma rays or electrons. More rarely, neutrons or protons are used. The dose given is prescribed in units of Gray, which is a measure of the amount of energy deposited in the tissue. A radical course of external beam radiotherapy for epithelial tumours delivers a dose between 50 and 70 Gray over 3–7 weeks using daily treatments of 1.6–2.5 Gray. Lymphomas and seminomas are relatively radiosensitive and can be treated with lower doses of 30–40 Gray. Palliative radiotherapy is given in significantly lower doses in schedules varying between one and ten treatments.

X-rays
  Superficial X-rays (80–140 kV)
  Deep X-rays (200–300 kV energy, sometimes termed orthovoltage X-rays)
  Supervoltage or megavoltage X-rays (2–20 MV and above, but usually in the range
    of 4–8 MV)
Radioisotopes
  Alpha-rays (of little value)
  Beta-rays (more penetrating, and of value for superficial areas)
  Gamma rays:
    small sealed sources, e.g. caesium-137 and iridium-192
    high-activity sources, for external beam treatment (so-called teletherapy sources)
Particulate beams of high energy
  Electrons
  Neutrons
  Protons

Table 4.1:   Radiations used in the treatment of cancer

External beam therapy

External beam radiotherapy is usually delivered using a linear accelerator which
generates X-rays of energies between 4 and 10 MV. The use of these machines
permits the administration of high doses to deep-seated tumours whilst minimizing the doses to skin and subcutaneous tissue, preventing the 'burns' seen
in the past. Linear accelerators also generate electrons, which may be used for
superficial tumours. Their physical properties allow the radiotherapist to spare
deeper sensitive structures accurately. Low-energy orthovoltage X-rays are used
in the treatment of skin cancers and in the palliation of superficial locally
recurrent or metastatic lesions.

Techniques of radiation beam therapy

Beams of X-rays or gamma-rays may be applied as a single direct beam, as an
opposed pair of beams either tangentially to, or directly through, the tissues to
be irradiated, or as multiple beams all convergent upon the volume to be
irradiated.

Accurate application of beams

When a limited deeply situated volume is to be treated, for example a carcinoma
of the middle third of the oesophagus or a carcinoma of the bladder, multiple

beams of radiation all directed at the required high-dose volume are needed. This requires precise application of beams.

CT scanning has proved to be of immense value in visualizing the limits of tumour volumes, and not infrequently indicates wider limits than those assessed from other investigations. Furthermore, facilities are now available for superimposing on the images of a CT scan picture the positions of radiation beams and the resulting dose distribution.

Brachytherapy

The dose received from a radioactive source falls off as the square of the distance from the source. Where it is possible to insert a radioactive source into or close to a tumour, therefore, high doses are received by the tumour with relative sparing of nearby normal tissues. Caesium-137, iridium-192 and iodine-125 are the most commonly used solid radioactive sources for this purpose. Caesium-137 is most commonly used as intracavitary therapy for the treatment of gynaecological malignancy such as cervical cancer. Iridium-192 is most commonly used as interstitial therapy, where pins or wires are temporarily inserted deep into the tumour.

Radioactive isotopes may be given orally or systemically where they are preferentially taken up by target tissue. The most common example of this is the use of iodine-131 in the treatment of differentiated thyroid tumours. Strontium-89 is taken up preferentially by the skeleton and may be used in the palliation of bone metastasis from, for example, carcinoma of the prostate. Other newer agents are being investigated and it may be possible in future to radiolabel specific anti-tumour antibodies to target radiotherapy more accurately.

Afterloading

Afterloading techniques
The handling of sealed sources of radiation for interstitial or intracavitary therapy exposes the operator and other staff in close proximity to a relatively small but finite radiation dose. Nevertheless, any reasonably obtained reduction in the exposure of staff to irradiation is to be commended and with this aim afterloading techniques have been developed. These require the insertion of applicator holders into the area to be treated, for example the vagina, uterine cavitary, side of tongue or tissues of the chest wall. Radio-opaque dummy sources are then inserted, the positions are checked radiologically and modified if necessary, and then the dummy sources are replaced by active ones.

Over the last 20 years better techniques of delivery of solid radioisotopes have reduced the unnecessary exposure experienced by the staff caring for these patients. Programmable afterloading systems such as the selectron and micro-selectron also permit the radiotherapist to tailor the dose delivered to an individual tumour.

Other modalities

The use of neutrons and protons for the therapy of advanced cancers has had a vogue. The results of most clinical studies have not suggested a routine role for these particles.

Total body irradiation may be used to sterilize bone marrow and tumour cells prior to bone marrow transplantation for leukaemia or chemosensitive tumours. Electrons may occasionally be used to treat the whole body in mycosis fungoides. Hemibody irradiation is a useful palliative measure for patients with widespread bony metastasis.

Uses of radiotherapy

Radical treatment
Radiotherapy may be used on its own or in combination with surgery and/or chemotherapy to provide local cure of many cancers. Its principal advantage over surgery is in the preservation of the structure and function of treated organs. Radiotherapy is particularly effective where the tumour burden is relatively small. It is often the case in these situations that the cure rates achieved with surgery and radiotherapy are comparable. In these situations radiotherapy is chosen where the functional or cosmetic result is likely to be better.

Radiosensitivity of tumours
The differing degrees of sensitivity to radiation damage shown by the cells of different tumours makes it possible to divide them broadly into three groups, termed 'radiosensitive', 'limited sensitivity' and 'radioresistant'. These terms are not absolute, however, as there is some variation within each group, and some degree of overlap between the groups. Nevertheless, the subdivisions in Table 4.2 are useful.

In general the radiosensitive tumours respond well to radiotherapy, and localized disease may be cured by appropriate doses of radiation alone. In more bulky stages, such as Hodgkin's disease, localized radiotherapy may be combined with chemotherapy to optimize tumour control.

Radiosensitive tumours
  Malignant lymphomas
  Seminoma of the testis
  Medulloblastoma, neuroblastoma, Wilms' tumour (nephroblastoma)
Tumours of limited sensitivity
  Squamous cell and basal cell carcinomas of the skin
  Squamous carcinoma of the head and neck
  Carcinoma of the bladder
  Squamous cancer of the cervix
Radioresistant tumours
  Osteosarcoma
  Malignant melanoma
  Large bowel adenocarcinomas
  Gliomas

Table 4.2:   Examples of the radiosensitivity of tumours

Tumours of limited sensitivity

The term 'tumours of limited sensitivity' is a useful one. The total dose of radiation tolerated by normal tissues decreases as the volume irradiated increases. The tumours in this group are sufficiently sensitive to be curable in many cases if the volume to be irradiated is small and tolerance high, but not so if the volume is larger and tolerance correspondingly lower. An example is that of an early localized carcinoma in the tonsillar region of the mouth, which has a curability rate of about 75%, compared with a more advanced local lesion with inoperable lymph node deposits in the neck, which is curable in only a few instances.

Radioresistant tumours

Tumours in the radioresistant group show some slight variations in their level of response to irradiation, but in general all would require doses in excess of local tissue tolerances to produce any significant response. Therefore they cannot be eradicated by this form of treatment. Surgical excision, if possible, offers the only chance of cure. Nevertheless, some show partial responses to irradiation, and this form of treatment can offer useful palliation of otherwise untreatable malignancies in carefully selected cases.

Side effects of radiotherapy

The damaging effects of radiation are induced in normal as well as abnormal tissues. Under favourable circumstances these effects can be lethal to tumour cells and sublethal to normal cells, so that the tumour cells are killed whereas the normal cells can recover. However, all normal tissues have a level of damage beyond which recovery does not occur; this is termed the 'tolerance dose'.

The dose of radiation which can be delivered is limited by immediate (but usually reversible) toxicity on rapidly dividing tissues such as the bowel, mucosa and skin, and by later irreversible organ damage. The known tolerance of vital organs is usually not exceeded and the incidence of late organ damage is less than 5% (for instance in the skin and bowel mucosa) and often less than 1% (e.g. in the brain or spinal cord). Early effects of radiation develop during treatment and usually settle within a month of its completion. They include mucositis, diarrhoea, proctitis, cystitis, skin erythema and hair loss. These effects are treated symptomatically. General malaise is a common feature of protracted treatment and can be alleviated by rest, understanding and support. The late carcinogenic effect of radiation manifests itself 10–20 years after treatment, with an increased incidence of second solid tumours. This risk is far outweighed by the benefit of the curative effects of radiotherapy.

Future developments

Hypoxia
The efficacy of radiation therapy is impaired by the presence of hypoxia in the tumour environment. A number of efforts have been made to improve this situation including the use of radiosensitizers and hyperbaric oxygen. The results so far have been disappointing, but there are hopes that a combination of breathing carbogen and the administration of nicotinamide may overcome both acute and chronic hypoxia and provide some therapeutic gain.

Radiosensitizers
There have been many reports of investigations into the radiosensitizing effects of so-called electron-affinic agents on hypoxic cells. These agents appear to mimic the radiobiological action of oxygen without being metabolized. They can diffuse into avascular areas.

A number of agents have been investigated, including misonidazole. Unfortunately, no definite clinical benefit has been achieved and as yet they have not entered routine clinical practice.

Fractionation
Recent evidence has suggested that the potential doubling time of tumours is rather shorter than previously believed. Multicentred international randomized trials are currently investigating the use of shortened fractionation schedules

designed to overcome tumour re-population during treatment. The shortest of these is the so-called CHART (continuous hyperfractionated accelerated radiotherapy) schedule in which treatment is completed within 12 days. Results from this study suggest an advantage in terms of local control in advanced head and neck cancers and an increase in survival of patients with lung cancer treated with this schedule.

Conformal therapy

The use of CT scans and fast computer systems now permits radiotherapists to visualize patient and tumour anatomy in three dimensions. Using this information and devices which customize the beam shape, treatments can for the first time be tailored to individual patients. Future research will help determine whether this 'conformal therapy' can reduce treatment toxicity and increase cure rates.

Cytotoxic chemotherapy

The great surgeon Bilroth first used chemotherapy in the form of arsenic in an attempt to cure his patients with lymphoma, but it was not until the First World War that the effects of mustard gas on bone marrow cells were reported and responses of lymphoma to nitrogen mustard observed.

Although enormous advances have been made in the treatment of cancer with chemotherapy over the past 40 years, it is obvious that cure is unusual and largely confined to a few relatively uncommon malignancies which generally affect the young. The chemotherapy here is given with *curative* intent. The common solid cancers in middle to old age have not responded as favourably to cytotoxic chemotherapy and, even though worthwhile remissions can be obtained with relief of symptoms and sometimes apparent disappearance of the tumour, the disease inevitably returns and the patient ultimately dies. In this situation the chemotherapy is given with *palliative* intent.

The effectiveness of chemotherapy ranges from almost always curative, as in gestational trophoblastic disease, through to rarely if ever achieving even a temporary response. Table 4.3 classifies tumours according to their clinical responsiveness to cytotoxic chemotherapy.

The tumour burden in a patient with advanced malignancy is in the range of 10^9–10^{11} cells. A treatment which destroys 99.9% of a tumour from a starting level of 10^9 cells would reduce the tumour load to 10^8 cells, enough to make the disease disappear, but clearly insufficient for cure. Repeated cycles of treatment

Curable	Highly responsive	Moderately responsive	Minimally responsive
Hodgkin's disease	Small-cell lung cancer	Colorectal	Pancreas
High-grade non-Hodgkin's lymphoma	Breast	Gastric	Kidney
Acute lymphoblastic leukaemia	Ovarian	Cervix	Brain
Acute myeloid leukaemia	Low-grade non-Hodgkin's lymphoma	Soft-tissue sarcoma	Oesophagus
Testicular tumours	Chronic myeloid leukaemia	Non-small-cell lung cancer	Hepatobiliary
Childhood malignancies	Multiple myeloma	Head and neck	
Gestational trophoblastic disease	Bone sarcomas	Bladder, melanoma, endometrium, prostate	

Table 4.3:   Responsiveness of advanced disseminated malignancy to chemotherapy

of this efficiency may reduce the tumour burden further, below the cure threshold where the body's own immune mechanisms can cope with the residuum, but more typically there exists a small proportion of resistant cells which repopulate the tumour, or drug resistance develops through genetic mutation in response to repeated sublethal exposure to cytotoxic agents.

It follows that chemotherapy is more likely to be effective if the tumour burden is low. This is the case in adjuvant chemotherapy given in certain clinical situations (e.g. following potentially curative surgery for breast or colon carcinoma) where there is no clinically detectable cancer left but a strong possibility of 'micro-metastases' exists, which if left untreated may give rise to overt tumour recurrence later.

Administration of chemotherapy

Initially cytotoxic drugs were given singly in relatively low doses and often continuously until tumour response was obtained. However, we now know this may promote the development of drug resistance, cause permanent damage to normal stem cells and does not take account of the rules of cell cycle kinetics. Although this form of therapy is still appropriate for some tumours it is more usual to use pulsed combination chemotherapy (Table 4.4).

Acronym	Cancer	Combination regimen
CMF	Breast cancer	Cyclophosphamide, Methotrexate, Fluorouracil
BEP	Testicular cancer	Bleomycin, Etoposide, cisPlatin
ACE	Small-cell lung cancer	Adriamycin (doxorubicin), Cyclophosphamide, Etoposide
CHOP	Non-Hodgkin's lymphoma	Cyclophosphamide, Hydroxydaunorubicin (doxorubicin), Oncovin (vincristine), Prednisolone

Table 4.4: Commonly used combination regimens

Using cytotoxic drugs in combination gives three major advantages:

1 Drugs with known effectiveness as single agents in treating a particular tumour but with different mechanisms of action can be used with synergistic effects.

2 Drugs of different toxicities can be used to avoid cumulative adverse effects.

3 Using more than one drug in a regimen may lessen the chance of resistance to the chemotherapy regimen.

Combination chemotherapy is usually given at 3–4-week intervals to allow normal tissue and bone marrow recovery. Some regrowth of the tumour population may occur, but in general tumour repopulation is slower and less efficient than for the normal cells.

Principles of cytotoxic activity

Chemotherapy drugs are rarely (if ever) entirely selective for cancer cells, and they also affect the normal cells which are taking part in the normal cell cycle. Some cytotoxic drugs may act at different phases of the cell cycle (phase-specific), such as those acting on synthesis of DNA or preventing spindle formation, while others act throughout the cell cycle (cycle-specific). Most drugs in fact fall into the latter group and will affect cells wherever they are in the cell cycle. In general cytotoxic drugs, unlike irradiation, will not affect cells in the resting G_0 phase. Clearly tumours with a higher proportion of cells in cycle are more likely to show response to chemotherapy than very slow-growing tumours with only a small growth fraction.

The optimum time to stop treatment remains undefined and is largely based on intuitive or empirical decisions. Nevertheless, there are very few circumstances where continuing chemotherapy for more than six cycles seems to have any effect on either the cure rate or prognosis.

In many situations the proportion of tumour cells in cycle is relatively small compared with the normal proliferating tissues of the bone marrow, skin and gastrointestinal tract. However, normal cells – particularly the stem cell population – are fortunately intrinsically less sensitive to chemotherapy and far more efficient at repairing drug-induced DNA damage than the cancer cell.

The time between treatments is important: if too short the normal stem cells will not recover adequately and cumulative toxicity will result, preventing or seriously delaying further cycles. If, on the other hand, the interval between courses is too long, tumour cell recovery will be risked, allowing regrowth or the development of drug resistance to occur.

In the clinic the appropriate time for retreatment is judged on the blood count. If the white blood cell and platelet counts have recovered to $>3.0 \times 10^9/L$ and $>100 \times 10^9/L$, respectively, full dose retreatment can proceed. Today, with the advent of bone marrow growth factors, it is possible to shorten the interval between chemotherapy treatments without prejudicing bone marrow stem cells. The clinical utility of this accelerated chemotherapy approach is a current area of intense investigation.

For many drugs the schedule of administration is important. Prolonged infusion of fluorouracil improves its therapeutic efficacy, while drugs such as etoposide are more effective when given in smaller doses over several days than when given as a large dose on a single day.

Biochemical classifications of cytotoxic drugs (Table 4.5)

The interaction of cancer chemotherapy agents upon cancer cell proliferation can be broadly classified into five main groups.

Alkylating agents	Mustine, cyclophosphamide, ifosfamide, chlorambucil
Antimetabolites	Methotrexate, fluorouracil, cytarabine, mercaptopurine
Intercalating agents	Doxorubicin, epirubicin, dactinomycin, bleomycin
Spindle poisons	Vincristine, vinblastine, paclitaxel
Miscellaneous drugs	Cisplatin, carboplatin, etoposide, mitozantrone

Table 4.5:   Examples of commonly used cytotoxic drugs

Alkylating agents
The main chemical reaction in this group of drugs is the formation of a covalent bond between highly reactive alkyl groups of the drug and the DNA double-stranded base pairs.

Antimetabolites
These drugs inhibit DNA synthesis by interfering with the incorporation of nucleic acid bases (cytosine, thiamine, adenine and guanine).

Intercalating agents
Like alkylating agents these drugs also form cross-strands in the DNA molecule but bind between the base pairs, either between the two strands or within a single strand, preventing cell division and precipitating fragmentation of the DNA chains.

Spindle poisons
The traditional drugs in this group are the vinca alkaloids, which are toxic to the microtubules of the mitotic spindle, a structure which is essential for the sorting and moving of chromosomes during mitosis. Mitosis is halted in metaphase.

Miscellaneous drugs
This group contains an ever-increasing number of agents with varying, sometimes unknown, mechanisms of action.

Drug resistance

The development of drug resistance is a complex phenomenon. The schedule of treatment may be wrong so that either regrowth of the tumour is occurring, or the exposure to a phase-specific drug is too short to affect more than a small percentage of the tumour cell population.

Clinically it is very clear that there is a lot of cross-resistance between chemotherapy drugs and that second-line therapy will only occasionally salvage a patient with a potentially curable cancer such as lymphoma or testicular teratoma, while in the palliative setting the benefits of second-line chemotherapy are marginal and often disputed.

Side effects of chemotherapy

Some side effects (such as myelosuppression) are seen with most drugs, whilst others are unique to individual drugs (for example cardiotoxicity with doxorubicin and related anthracyclines). For certain drugs, particularly cisplatin, methotrexate and ifosfamide, renal function must also be carefully checked prior to administration.

Myelosuppression and immunosuppression

The patient with widespread malignant disease may have suppression of bone marrow function and the lymphoreticular system before treatment is started. Cytotoxic chemotherapy initially will worsen the situation in such cases. Great caution is needed to avoid the possibility of overwhelming infection; regular checking of the blood count may be indicated and any infection must be treated early and aggressively. Most infections come from endogenous organisms, particularly the patient's own gut flora, and sensible hygiene precautions and good hand-washing are usually sufficient.

Thrombocytopenia is a less common problem with solid tumour chemotherapy but is a life-threatening toxicity of treatments for leukaemia, with haemorrhage becoming increasingly likely as the platelet count falls below 20×10^9/L. Anaemia is more of a long-term complication of myelosuppression and many patients require a blood transfusion at some time during chemotherapy.

Recently, bone marrow growth factors such as filgrastim and lenograstim (granulocyte colony-stimulating factors) and molgramostim (granulocyte macrophage colony-stimulating factor) have been introduced into cancer care. These natural substances stimulate the development and maturation of bone marrow progenitor cells, particularly of the white cell series. Administration of bone marrow growth factors both shortens the duration and reduces the severity of chemotherapy-induced neutropenia. This reduces the risk of severe infection and enables the delivery of high doses of chemotherapy at more frequent intervals.

In some clinical situations bone marrow stem cells, harvested either from the bone marrow itself or from the peripheral blood after stimulation with chemotherapy and growth factors, can be collected to support the administration of high-dose chemotherapy. Cells are removed from the patient, then cryopreserved until after high-dose chemotherapy, with or without whole-body irradiation, has been administered. Once the drugs have been metabolized, the cells are re-infused and bone marrow function returns after 7–21 days.

Gastrointestinal side effects

Nausea and vomiting are common side effects which in the past were often difficult to control and occasionally led to poor treatment compliance. The introduction of combination anti-emetic regimens and new specific anti-emetics now enables excellent control of acute (first 24 hours) control of emesis with even the most toxic agents, such as cisplatin. For drugs known to be severely emetogenic, a combination of a $5HT_3$ antagonist such as granisetron or ondansetron plus a corticosteroid is recommended, while for moderately emetogenic agents traditional drugs such as metoclopramide, domperidone, haloperidol and prochlorperazine are usually sufficient.

Delayed emesis is a particular problem of treatment with cisplatin, with symptoms persisting for several days. The underlying mechanisms are more complex and treatments less effective. Metoclopramide and dexamethasone are the best currently available agents for this type of chemotherapy-induced emesis. Anticipatory emesis is a conditioned response to previous unpleasant chemotherapy which also requires a different treatment approach, anxiolytics and behavioural therapy being the most widely tested.

Diarrhoea is occasionally a problem, particularly with drugs such as fluorouracil, but severe toxicity to the small and large bowel is extremely uncommon and symptomatic treatment is usually very effective.

Germinal cell effects

Contraception is very important during cytotoxic chemotherapy as many of the cytotoxic drugs are teratogenic and mutagenic. Fetal conception during cytotoxic chemotherapy may result in abortion of the embryo, or in gross congenital abnormalities of the fetus. If chemotherapy has to be given during early pregnancy, termination is usually recommended.

Infertility may occur after cytotoxic chemotherapy. It is particularly a feature of high-dose alkylating agents. In women this is accompanied by early menopause, while in men endocrine function is generally preserved, although sperm production is ablated. Infertility is most likely in those treated during puberty and in older patients, particularly women nearing the menopause. For men, sperm storage is now available in most centres. However, cryopreservation of ova or ovaries is not generally available. Recovery of germinal epithelium is often slow and fertility may not return for months or even years after completing chemotherapy.

If fertility is at all a possibility, the patient should be advised to avoid conception for at least a year after completion of chemotherapy. To date, the children conceived by parents who have had previous chemotherapy have shown no increased evidence of congenital abnormalities or subsequent malignant disease.

Less frequent side effects

Cardiomyopathy, or overt heart failure, is a dose-related adverse effect of anthracycline treatment. It is more likely in patients who are also receiving cardiac irradiation or in those with a past history of cardiac disease. As the dose of anthracycline increases, monitoring of ventricular function by echocardiography or radionuclide angiography is recommended.

Occasionally chemotherapy will cause lung damage. Diffuse alveolar damage, which may progress to fatal pulmonary fibrosis, is seen with high doses of bleomycin. Mitomycin, busulphan and certain other alkylating agents also occasionally cause respiratory problems.

Hepatotoxicity is an occasional side-effect. It usually takes the form of hepatocellular damage and may manifest as disordered liver function tests or jaundice. Long-term exposure to methotrexate is the best-described cause. In addition, veno-occlusive disease of the liver may accompany high-dose intensive chemotherapy.

Nephrotoxicity is a common complication of treatment with cisplatin, and great care should be taken to ensure adequate hydration of patients during therapy. Some degree of tubular damage is almost inevitable, with loss of magnesium, calcium and potassium. Tubular damage may also be seen after treatment with methotrexate or ifosfamide. Methotrexate-induced renal damage is reduced by alkalinization of the urine, while careful intravenous hydration and co-administration of mesna reduces the risk of ifosfamide-induced damage.

Neurotoxicity (which may affect peripheral, autonomic and cranial nerves) is most commonly seen with the vinca-alkaloids, particularly vincristine and with cisplatin. Ototoxicity is another important toxicity of cisplatin, affecting particularly the appreciation of high-frequency tones.

Special precautions

Drug dosages are usually based on the surface area of the patient. In patients with impaired renal or hepatic function the doses of certain drugs excreted by the kidney or metabolized and excreted by the liver will have to be reduced. This information must always be checked in the relevant drug data sheet.

Other treatments

Immunotherapy

Immunotherapy in the patient with cancer aims at stimulating the cell-mediated, humoral and phagocytic systems on the assumption that the normal immunological mechanisms have been unable to deal with the growing tumour. Evidence suggests that a powerful immunological reaction is necessary to destroy even a small number of malignant cells; the critical range of tumour cell acceptance or rejection seems to be 10^5–10^7 depending on the immunological state of the host. For malignant disease to become evident, 10^8 cells are required; it follows that effective immunotherapy must depend on surgery, chemotherapy and radiotherapy for reducing the tumour burden to the minimum number of cells.

Immunostimulation holds exciting promise in the field of cancer therapy but has been bedevilled by the lack of controlled clinical trials. An example of this is the wide publicity given to the antiviral agent interferon; this acts, probably via the immune system, as an anti-cancer agent but is as yet of unproven clinical value. Immunotherapy is not without adverse effects and cannot yet replace the standard treatments of surgery, radiation and cytotoxic drugs; generally it should be given only as an adjuvant after the removal of the bulk of the tumour by these other treatments.

One major advance in immunotherapy (perhaps now better termed biological response modifier therapy) is the development of new molecular biological techniques. In this 'recombinant technology', large amounts of rare polypeptides involved in immune regulation can be produced by gene cloning and subsequent expression in tissue culture cells or micro-organisms. Immune regulators, for example interferon and interleukins, produced in this way are currently being studied in clinical trials. The identification of human tumour-associated antigens which promote cytotoxic T-lymphocyte anti-tumour activity has provided us with the opportunity to develop vaccines and therefore opened up exciting new possibilities for cancer therapy.

Endocrine therapy

In 1896, the Scottish surgeon Beatson demonstrated that oophorectomy can cause regression of metastatic breast carcinoma. It has since become apparent that the growth of some tumours is hormone-dependent and that changing the balance of the hormonal environment can lead to regression of such tumours. A summary of the various endocrine procedures used in cancer therapy and some of the side effects is given in Tables 4.6 and 4.7.

Hormone therapy is rarely curative however, and often needs to be combined with other treatment modalities such as surgery, radiotherapy and chemotherapy. The recognition of the presence of hormonal receptors, particularly in breast cancer tissue, has made the use of endocrine treatment far less

Tumour	Therapy

Breast
  Premenopausal
  Perimenopausal
	Oophorectomy
	Anti-oestrogens
	Androgens
	Corticosteroids
	Anti-adrenals

Postmenopausal	Anti-oestrogens Oestrogens Progestogens
Male	Orchidectomy, oestrogens
Prostate	Orchidectomy, oestrogens Orchidectomy, gonadorelins Anti-androgens, oestrogens
Uterine body Kidney Haematological Thyroid	Progestogens Progestogens Corticosteroids Thyroxine

Table 4.6:   Examples of endocrine therapy for cancer

Therapy	Side effects
Oestrogens	Nausea, fluid retention, vaginal bleeding, feminization, hypercalcaemia
Androgens	Virilization, cholestatic jaundice
Anti-oestrogens	Nausea, skin rashes
Progestogens	Fluid retention, nausea
Corticosteroids	Fluid retention, hypertension, diabetes, osteoporosis, Cushingoid features, immunosuppression

Table 4.7:   Side effects of endocrine therapy

empirical, since detection of these receptors appears to be a reliable method of predicting hormonal responsiveness.

Hormone therapy is particularly valuable in breast cancer and prostate cancer. The use of the anti-oestrogen tamoxifen as an adjuvant has been proven to reduce the risk of relapse of breast cancer in postmenopausal patients. Its use for these patients is now routine. 75–80% of patients with metastatic or locally advanced prostate cancer will obtain rapid benefit from endocrine manoeuvres designed to reduce the androgen drive to the tumour. This may involve orchidectomy or the use of drugs such as cyproterone acetate or goserelin.

The role of steroids in cancer treatment deserves special consideration. Apart from their direct cytotoxic effect they have a role in the management of certain peripheral cancer effects. The physical and psychological well-being of a patient may be transiently improved, and hypercalcaemia and cerebral oedema (in association with brain metastases) may respond dramatically to prednisolone and dexamethasone respectively.

5

The management of common cancers

B W Hancock and R E Coleman

Lung cancer

Basic facts

The bronchial tree is the commonest site of human cancer. Its incidence has increased but may now be plateauing. It is commoner in men than in women by a ratio of about 2.5:1, though this difference is decreasing. The main aetiological factors are:

- smoking
- industrial exposure to dust and chemicals
- genetic susceptibility.

Pathology

75% of tumours arise in the main bronchi; the remainder are peripheral. Squamous carcinomas account for approximately 50% of tumours; small-cell undifferentiated (oat cell) carcinomas about 25%; the remaining tumours are adenocarcinomas (15%) and large-cell carcinomas (10%). Local spread is to adjacent structures (chest wall, mediastinum, pericardium, pleura and diaphragm); lymphatic spread is to the regional nodes, particularly those in the mediastinum and lower neck; blood spread most commonly results in metastases to bones, brain and liver, although any organ may be involved.

Clinical features

Symptoms and signs therefore arise from:

- the primary tumour itself
  - haemoptysis
  - cough
  - wheeze and stridor
  - dyspnoea
  - infection

- local extension of the primary tumour
  - pain
  - dyspnoea from pleural effusion
  - cardiac symptoms from pericardial involvement

- lymphatic spread to regional nodes
  - lymphadenopathy
  - superior vena caval obstruction
  - dysphagia
  - left recurrent nerve palsy
  - phrenic nerve paralysis
  - sympathetic nerve paralysis (Horner's syndrome)
  - brachial plexus involvement (Pancoast's syndrome)
  - lymphatic obstruction with pleural effusion

- bloodstream spread
  - bone pain
  - personality change or other evidence of brain metastases
  - hepatomegaly (often painful) and jaundice
  - spinal cord compression

- paraneoplastic syndromes
  - systemic (anorexia/cachexia, fever)
  - endocrine (ectopic hormone secretion, hypercalcaemia)
  - skeletal (clubbing, hypertrophic pulmonary osteoarthropathy)
  - neurological (cerebellar ataxia, peripheral neuropathy)
  - haematological (anaemia, coagulopathies)
  - dermatological (ichthyosis, pruritus).

Investigations

After chest X-ray (and in certain cases computerized tomography) a pathological diagnosis is mandatory. Sometimes this is established from sputum cytology. More often, fibreoptic bronchoscopic biopsy is needed and occasionally, for peripheral lesions, guided needle biopsy or even open operation may be required.

Treatment

Surgery is only possible in a minority of patients but it offers the best hope of cure in localized tumours.

Radiotherapy may be appropriate in localized tumours where surgery is declined or the patient is unfit. Obviously radical treatment is appropriate for only the minority of patients with localized disease in the bronchus and adjacent lymph nodes. Radiotherapy is the mainstay of symptom palliation.

Palliative care is very important in lung cancer – communication is just as vitally important as the relief of psychological and physical symptoms.

Cytotoxic chemotherapy has a major role in the treatment of small-cell lung cancer; it may even cure a small number of patients. Drugs such as vincristine, doxorubicin, epirubicin, cyclophosphamide, ifosfamide, cisplatin and etoposide are often used in combinations of two or more. The role of chemotherapy in non-small-cell lung cancer is still being evaluated in clinical trials.

Prognosis

The final results of treatment of lung cancer are very poor. About 80% of patients are dead within one year; the overall five-year survival is still only about 5%. In limited-stage small-cell lung cancer, chemotherapy improves average survival prospects from six months to over a year; in more extensive disease, median survival may be prolonged from a few weeks to a few months.

Breast

Basic facts

About one in 12 women will develop breast cancer at some time in their life and there is likely to be a modest increase in incidence and mortality. Breast carcinomas are often metastatic at a very early stage in their development; as a result not more than 30% of patients are presently 'curable'. However, there is a very long natural history (about two-thirds are alive at five years) and many patients live for several years; their care accounts for a major proportion of any oncology workload. Appropriate mammography to screen for early cancers or pre-cancerous abnormalities could reduce the mortality in those screened by up to a third. The main aetiological factors are:

- genetic susceptibility

- hormone status – menarche, menopause, age of first child

- high animal-fat diet.

Pathology

Virtually all breast cancers are adenocarcinoma and the majority are ductal (80%); the other major pattern is lobular, in which bilateral tumours are more frequent. Rare types are tubular, medullary and colloid. Carcinomas may be in situ or invasive (infiltrating). Breast cancer spreads by local infiltration into skin and chest wall, via lymphatics to regional lymph nodes and via the bloodstream to any distant organ but particularly the bones, lungs, liver and brain.

Clinical features

Symptoms and signs therefore arise from:

- the primary tumour itself
  – breast lump(s)

- local extension of the primary tumour
  – breast abnormalities (peau d'orange, inflammation or ulceration, affecting the skin, or Paget's disease, affecting the nipple)

- lymphatic spread to regional nodes and the other breast
  – lymphadenopathy
  – breast lump(s)

- bloodstream spread
  – bone pain, pathological fractures, spinal cord compression
  – dyspnoea (pleural effusion, lung deposits)
  – hepatomegaly and jaundice
  – personality change or other evidence of brain metastasis

- paraneoplastic syndromes
  – hypercalcaemia.

Investigations

Histological confirmation is mandatory, usually by fine needle aspiration or Trucut needle biopsy; however, surgical excision of a suspicious lump may be necessary. The disease may be staged simplistically into three categories — operable, locally advanced and metastatic. A number of investigations may be performed to evaluate staging; various scans may be required for patients with large, locally advanced or metastatic cancer.

Treatment

Surgery is the cornerstone in the treatment of operable cancer. Debate over the need for mastectomy continues but the recent consensus is that more limited surgery may be safely employed, though the views of the patient are highly relevant here. Axillary node sampling and/or clearance is usually undertaken. Surgery may also be cosmetic (e.g. late breast reconstruction after mastectomy) or palliative (in advanced loco-regional disease).

Radiotherapy is usually given as an adjuvant to surgery to reduce local recurrence after local surgical procedures, and after mastectomy where the tumour is large or semifixed or where the axillary nodes are involved. Radiotherapy has a major role in palliation.

Endocrine therapy may be adjuvant or palliative. Adjuvant tamoxifen therapy increases survival in postmenopausal patients; in premenopausal patients its role and that of ovarian ablation are still being studied in clinical trials.

In advanced breast cancer about one third of tumours are hormone-responsive. Tamoxifen is the preferred first line of treatment in postmenopausal women; second-line agents include the progestogens — medroxyprogesterone acetate and megestrol are often favoured for their safety and simplicity — and aminoglutethimide (which inhibits the conversion of androgens to oestrogens in the peripheral tissues) with steroid replacement. Options for premenopausal women include an artificial menopause by oophorectomy, irradiation or gonadotrophin-releasing hormone agonists, or tamoxifen. Hardly ever used nowadays are oestrogens, androgens, adrenalectomy and hypophysectomy.

About one-third of patients showing response to one type of hormone therapy will respond to a second agent.

Chemotherapy may also be adjuvant or palliative. The place of adjuvant chemotherapy is becoming clearer: in premenopausal patients the chances of dying from the disease five years after diagnosis are reduced by about 30%. Cyclophosphamide, methotrexate and fluorouracil (CMF), in combination, are the drugs most often used.

In advanced disease, single agents (such as doxorubicin or epirubicin) or combination chemotherapy (with two or more of drugs such as cyclo-phosphamide, methotrexate, fluorouracil, mitozantrone, mitomycin, vincristine, doxorubicin or epirubicin) produce responses and effective palliation in up to half of patients treated. Responses are often short, though durable remissions are sometimes seen.

Prognosis

A number of factors have prognostic importance:

- tumour size

- presence of axillary lymph node involvement

- histological type and grade

- steroid receptor expression

- various biological indices of cell proliferation and oncogene expression.

The most important prognostic factor is axillary lymph node involvement, the prognosis deteriorating as the number of involved lymph nodes increases.

As already indicated breast carcinomas are often metastatic (at a microscopic level) at a very early stage in their development; as a result of this only about 30% of patients are currently curable — by appropriate surgery with or without adjuvant therapy. The natural history is very long and over 60% of patients are alive at five years. Once breast cancer has become metastatic, the median survival is 24 months; the clinical course and pattern of metastasis are, however, very variable, some patients deteriorating very rapidly, others sustaining a good quality of life with indolent disease over many years.

Alimentary tract

Oesophagus

Basic facts
Malignant tumours of the oesophagus represent about 5% of all cancers; they occur mainly in later life and are commoner in males than females. The main aetiological factors are:

- smoking

- alcohol consumption

- disorders of oesophageal motility

- chronic acid reflux.

Histological features
The majority of oesophageal tumours are squamous cell carcinomas, arising in stratified epithelium. Adenocarcinomas account for about 15% of lesions and may arise at the lower end in gastric-type mucosa which can extend a short distance up into the oesophagus. Tumours arise most often at one of the areas of partial natural narrowing: the pharyngo-oesophageal junction (one-fifth), the junction of the upper and middle thirds, where it is crossed by the left main bronchus (two-fifths), and the lower end where the oesophagus passes through the diaphragm (two-fifths). Local infiltration occurs early (circumferentially and longitudinally) and invasion of adjacent mediastinal structures may occur. Lymphatic spread is to mediastinal, neck and upper abdominal nodes. Distant blood-borne metastasis is mainly to the liver through the portal venous system, but also to the lungs and bones.

Clinical features
Symptoms and signs therefore arise from:

- the primary tumour itself
  – dysphagia

- local extension of the primary tumour
  – dysphagia
  – retrosternal pain
  – weight loss (reduced food intake)

- lymphatic spread to regional nodes
  – lymphadenopathy of the mediastinum or neck

- bloodstream spread
  – hepatomegaly and jaundice
  – dyspnoea (lung metastases)
  – bone pain.

Investigations
The most valuable investigations are radiology (barium swallow) and endoscopy (oesophagoscopy), where biopsy can be taken and the lumen dilated if necessary. Other investigations, for example chest CT scan, may be necessary to assess the extent of the lesion and resectability.

Treatment

Surgery is appropriate for middle- and lower-third tumours and is the only potentially curative treatment. For upper-third tumours surgical clearance and reconstruction are often impossible.

Radiotherapy is the treatment of choice therefore for tumours of the oesophagus. Palliative radiotherapy should be considered for patients with more extensive lesions, particularly for the relief of dysphagia. Palliation can also be achieved, sometimes with less upset, by endoscopic dilatation of the malignant stricture, particularly if combined with the insertion of a plastic endoprosthesis (for example Celestin tube). Multidisciplinary supportive care is important to improve morale and quality of life.

Prognosis

The results of treatment are disappointing, with overall survival figures of about 20% at five years for upper-third tumours, 6% for middle-third lesions, and 15% for those in the lower-third.

Stomach

Basic facts

Gastric cancer is one of the commonest malignancies of western civilization; the highest incidence is in the sixth decade and the disease is twice as common in males as in females. The main aetiological factors are:

- dietary carcinogens

- smoking

- alcohol

- achlorhydria

- chronic reflux of bile salts

- blood group (O protective, increased incidence with A).

Pathology

The vast majority of gastric cancers are adenocarcinomas, which may be diffuse and infiltrating, fungating or ulcerated. The diffuse variety produces the classic 'leather bottle stomach' or linitis plastica. Local extension leads to invasion of adjacent structures. Lymphatic spread is early to local lymph nodes. Spread to the liver via the portal system is common, and transcoelomic spread may also occur.

Clinical features
Symptoms and signs therefore arise from:

- the primary tumour itself
  - dyspepsia
  - haematemesis
  - epigastric mass

- local extension of the primary tumour
  - pyloric obstruction

- lymphatic spread to regional nodes
  - lymphadenopathy (left supraclavicular node enlargement — 'Virchow's node', 'Troisier's sign'

- bloodstream spread
  - hepatomegaly and jaundice

- transcoelomic spread
  - ascites
  - ovarian deposits — Krukenberg tumors

- paraneoplastic syndromes
  - systemic features (weight loss, anorexia and anaemia).

Investigations
Barium meal and gastroscopy (with biopsy) are the most helpful investigations. Ultrasound or CT scanning of the liver are usually performed before surgery is undertaken.

Treatment
Surgery is the only radical treatment available, with excision of the stomach (gastrectomy) and adjacent lymph node groups. Radiotherapy has little to offer as radical treatment but may be useful in palliating pain. There is considerable interest in the use of chemotherapy, but it is still the subject of clinical trials.

Prognosis
Only about 25% of patients who undergo radical surgery are alive at five years. Many tumours are inoperable when diagnosed, with a median survival of

3–6 months. At present the only realistic hope of improving results lies in earlier diagnosis so that radical surgery is still possible.

Pancreas

Basic facts
Adenocarcinoma of the pancreas is a disease of later life affecting males slightly more frequently than females. The main aetiological factors are:

- smoking

- pancreatitis.

Pathology
90% of tumours arise from the ducts and 10% from the glandular elements and are almost invariably mucin-secreting adenocarcinomas. The tumour arises most often in the head of the organ and infiltrates through the gland or spreads along the pancreatic duct to the ampulla of Vater. Regional lymph node and portal venous spread occurs early; systemic bloodstream metastasis is usually to bone and/or lung.

Clinical features
Symptoms and signs therefore arise from:

- the primary tumour itself
  – jaundice
  – malabsorption/steatorrhoea

- local extension of the primary tumour
  – back pain

- lymphatic spread to regional nodes
  – portal obstruction

- bloodstream spread
  – hepatomegaly and jaundice

- paraneoplastic syndromes
  – coagulopathies (migrating thrombophlebitis and disseminated intravascular coagulation).

Investigations
Visualization of the pancreas is often difficult and this contributes to the typical delay in diagnosis. Histological confirmation is usually possible by percutaneous CT-guided biopsy or by endoscopy, though occasionally laparotomy is necessary.

Treatment
Surgery offers the only chance of radical treatment and only in a small number of patients. Palliative cholecystoduodenostomy for biliary drainage may be of benefit.

Radiotherapy and cytotoxic chemotherapy have very little part to play in treatment. Pain relief may require coeliac plexus block. A biliary stent quite often provides relief of obstructive jaundice and of the associated pruritus.

Prognosis
Operability rates are low and five-year survival figures quoted are less than 1%.

Colon/rectum

Basic facts
Cancer of the large bowel is common, and in white races accounts for more deaths than any other form of malignant disease. It occurs mainly in middle and old age, and affects males and females equally. The principal sites are the caecum and ascending colon (15%), rectosigmoid region (40%) and rectum (35%). The main aetiological factors are:

- single or multiple polyps

- long-standing ulcerative colitis

- low-residue diet

- genetic susceptibility.

Pathology
Colorectal tumours are adenocarcinomas (sometimes with mucin production), frequently staining for carcinoembryonic antigen (CEA). The tumour spreads circumferentially and longitudinally. Tumours may be of exophytic or ulcerative, infiltrative types. Lymph node and haematological spread are common, the latter mainly through the portal circulation to the liver.

Clinical features

Symptoms and signs therefore arise from:

- the primary tumour itself
  - blood/mucus in the faeces
  - change in bowel habit (alternating constipation and diarrhoea)
  - anaemia

- local extension of the primary tumour
  - pain on defecation
  - tenesmus
  - intestinal obstruction
  - intestinal perforation/peritonitis
  - fistulae (e.g. rectovesical)

- bloodstream spread
  - hepatomegaly and jaundice

- transcoelomic spread
  - ascites.

Investigations

Rectal tumours are often palpable on digital rectal examination and about three-quarters of colorectal tumours can be seen and biopsied by sigmoidoscopy. Colonoscopy and barium enema examination may be needed for more proximal tumours. Some form of liver imaging (ultrasound or CT) and a chest X-ray are usually performed before elective surgery. Colorectal tumours are staged according to Dukes' classification:

A confined to bowel wall

B invasion through the bowel wall

C regional lymph node involvement

D presence of metastases.

The majority of lesions are Dukes' B and C.

Treatment

Surgery is the only curative treatment — wide margin excision of the involved segment of bowel plus regional lymph nodes with end-to-end anastomosis. Tumours of the lower rectum may require abdominoperineal resection and colostomy. Palliative surgery may be required to bypass an obstruction or create a defunctioning colostomy to provide good relief of symptoms. Resection of liver metastases is also now possible.

Radiotherapy has a limited role in treating bowel tumours but given preoperatively increases the proportion of rectal tumours which become re-sectable, whilst postoperatively it may reduce local recurrence rates.

Adjuvant fluorouracil-based chemotherapy reduces the probability of re-currence after apparently curative surgery by about one-third; patients with Dukes' C disease are now increasingly being offered this routinely (though clinical trials continue to investigate if fluorouracil is best given with folinic acid or the immune stimulator levamisole, and for what duration). In the palliation of advanced disease over half of patients will show symptomatic response and over a third of tumours show objective responses to chemotherapy with fluorouracil (given either by continuous infusion, or in combination with the modulating activity of folinic acid).

Prognosis
With radical surgery, despite an 80% resection rate, almost half of patients will develop recurrent disease within two years, usually in the liver. The prognosis of colorectal cancer is most related to Dukes' stage. Reported five-year survival rates are 80% for Dukes' A, 60% for Dukes' B, 30% for Dukes' C and 5% for those with metastatic disease at presentation.

Gynaecological

Uterine cervix

Basic facts
Carcinoma of the cervix is one of the commonest malignancies in females, predominantly affecting women in their 50s and 60s but showing an increase in younger age groups. There is a wide geographical variation in incidence, with the highest levels being found in South America, where the incidence is ten times higher than in the UK. Screening by cervical cytology for pre-cancerous change (cervical intraepithelial neoplasia, CIN) can identify earlier those needing treatment; the incidence of invasive carcinoma may therefore be reduced by at least 20%. The main aetiological factors are:

• early first intercourse and first pregnancy

- multiple partners

- viral infection (herpes simplex, human papilloma virus)

- lower socio-economic groups.

Pathology
Over 90% of cancers are squamous cell carcinomas (from the vaginal cervix or endocervical canal epithelium); the rest are mostly adenocarcinomas arising from the endocervix. Invasive tumours may be exophytic or infiltrating and ulcerative. Local spread is to the upper vagina and the body of the uterus; lymphatic spread occurs early; blood-borne metastases (particularly to bones and lungs) are less common and in many cases the disease remains confined to the pelvis until very advanced.

Clinical features
Symptoms and signs therefore arise from:

- the primary tumour itself
  - abnormal cervical smear
  - bleeding/discharge

- local growth of the primary tumour
  - pain (pelvic nerve infiltration)
  - fistulae to the bladder or rectum
  - ureteric obstruction

- lymphatic spread to regional nodes
  - low back pain (para-aortic lymphadenopathy)

- bloodstream spread
  - pain (bone involvement)
  - breathlessness (lung involvement).

Investigations
Clinical assessment is mandatory and this will include examination under anaesthetic to assess local extension of the tumour. Various imaging techniques may also delineate the extent of pelvic disease. Cervical cancer is staged according to the FIGO system from stage 1 (basically disease confined to the cervix) through to stage 4 (involvement of bladder or rectum or distant metastases). Stages 2 and 3 depend on the amount of tumour extension to the vagina and/or pelvis.

Treatment

For disease confined to the cervix, radical radiotherapy and surgery are effective treatments. Radical surgery (Wertheim's hysterectomy) is usually the treatment of choice in young fit patients.

If radical radiotherapy is given this usually involves intracavitary treatment using an intrauterine and vaginal source (brachytherapy) together with external beam treatment. For tumours extending beyond the cervix (stages 2 and 3), radical radiotherapy is usually the treatment of choice; intracavitary and whole pelvic external beam therapy is given. For extensive pelvic disease or metastases (stage 4) treatment should be considered palliative. This may be radiotherapy for local advanced disease, palliative surgery where there is a fistula, or chemotherapy for relief of systemic symptoms.

Prognosis

The results of treatment are very much related to the presenting stage. Five-year survivals are about 80% for stage 1, 65% for stage 2, 25% for stage 3, and less than 5% for stage 4.

Endometrium

Basic facts

This tumour generally affects an older, predominantly postmenopausal group of women; its incidence is of the same order as cervical cancer. The main aetiological factors are:

- low parity
- obesity
- diabetes
- prolonged oestrogen stimulation
- (use of tamoxifen for breast cancer).

Pathology

Most are adenocarcinomas; pre-cancerous conditions include endometrial hyperplasia and polyps. Endometrial carcinoma tends to remain localized within the pelvis, with slow invasion of the myometrium followed by spread to the cervix, vagina and ovaries. Lymphatic and blood-borne metastases arise late.

Clinical features
Symptoms and signs therefore arise from:

- the primary tumour itself
  – postmenopausal bleeding

- local extension of the primary tumour
  – pelvic discomfort

- bloodstream spread
  – bone pain
  – dyspnoea from lung metastases.

Investigations
Histological diagnosis is usually made from uterine curettings or aspirates, and a CT scan may be done to assess local spread and lymph node status. Staging is by the FIGO classification — stage 1 (confined to the endometrium), stage 2 (invasion of the cervix), stage 3 (pelvic involvement), and stage 4 (bladder or rectum involvement or distant metastases).

Treatment
This tumour is generally managed by surgery with total abdominal hysterectomy and bilateral salpingo-oophorectomy.

Radiotherapy (brachytherapy) may be used in addition to surgery in some cases; in others (where the disease is more extensive) radical external beam radiotherapy plus intracavitary treatment may be given. Patients with locally advanced or metastatic tumours may show responses to progestogens (medroxyprogesterone acetate or megestrol).

Chemotherapy is not recommended.

Prognosis
The prognosis for endometrial carcinoma is generally good, with 85% five-year survival for stage 1 disease.

Ovary

Basic facts
Ovarian cancer tends to occur in women over the age of 40; it causes 4000 deaths each year in the UK. The main aetiological factors are:

- nulliparity

- higher socio-economic status.

Pathology
Most ovarian cancers are of an epithelial origin, and typically have a mixture of solid and cystic components, with the latter containing either serous or mucinous material. These tumours spread primarily by local extension and peritoneal seeding. Lymphatic spread is common and haematogenous spread may result in lung and liver metastases. Pleural effusions are quite common.

Clinical features
Symptoms and signs therefore arise from:

- the primary tumour itself
  – abdominal discomfort
  – palpable mass
  – urinary symptoms
  – bowel symptoms
  – backache

- lymphatic spread to regional nodes
  – cervical lymphadenopathy

- bloodstream spread
  – dyspnoea (pleural effusion)
  – hepatomegaly and jaundice.

Investigations
Histological diagnosis is usually made at operation. Imaging of the abdomen and pelvis (ultrasound/CT scan) may be performed. Serum CA125 is a useful blood marker for ovarian cancer: it is elevated in 80% of cases and is a useful monitor of response to treatment. Ovarian cancer is staged using the FIGO system: stage 1 confined to the ovary, stage 2 pelvic spread, stage 3 abdominal cavity spread and stage 4 distant metastases.

Treatment
Expert gynaecological surgery is essential; total abdominal hysterectomy, bilateral salpingo-oophorectomy and removal of the omentum should be performed and any metastases maximally debulked. The smaller the amount of residual disease remaining at the end of surgery, the better the prognosis. For stage 1 disease further 'adjuvant' therapy may be of benefit, and this is currently being tested in clinical trials.

For more advanced disease, chemotherapy is standard. Cisplatin or (more commonly these days) carboplatin are the usual drugs given, typically as single agents in the UK but as part of combination chemotherapy in other parts of the world. The response rate to such chemotherapy is over 60%. For elderly or frail patients single alkylating therapy can be used, although response rates are lower. Recently a new, highly active drug, paclitaxel (Taxol), has been shown to be effective in platinum-resistant advanced ovarian cancer; the role of this expensive new drug is being further evaluated in clinical studies.

Nowadays, radiotherapy is rarely indicated in the management of ovarian cancer.

Prognosis
Patients with stage 1 ovarian cancer have a good prognosis, with 80% five-year survival. For more advanced disease the results are poorer — only 30% at stage 3 and less than 5% of patients with stage 4 disease will survive five years.

Male genital tract

Testis

Basic facts
Testicular tumours account for only 1% of all cancers but are the commonest malignancy in young men aged 18–35. In the UK there are just over 1000 cases per year and the incidence is rising. There are two main types of testicular tumour: seminoma is the most common type accounting for a half of patients and with a peak incidence in the fourth decade of life, while teratomas account for a third of patients with a peak incidence in the third decade of life. Most of the remaining tumours are a mixture of both seminoma and teratoma. The main aetiological factor is developmental abnormality (testicular maldescent).

Pathology
Seminomas are solid tumours which are generally well circumscribed with a pale lobulated appearance, whereas teratomas are usually haemorrhagic and contain cysts.

Microscopically seminomas are fairly uniform tumours whereas teratomas may contain a range of cell types with varying differentiation; they may be completely undifferentiated or show features of either trophoblastic or yolk sac differentiation. Local invasion is into the tunica vaginalis and along the spermatic cord. Seminomas spread mainly via the lymphatic system to para-aortic and mediastinal lymph nodes, while teratomas tend to metastasize to both the lymph nodes and via the bloodstream, particularly to the lungs but also the liver and brain.

Clinical features
Symptoms and signs therefore arise from:

- the primary tumour itself
  - testicular swelling
  - testicular discomfort

- local extension of the primary tumour
  - groin and testicular pain

- lymphatic spread to the regional nodes
  - back pain (enlarged para-aortic nodes)
  - palpable abdominal mass

- bloodstream spread
  - haemoptysis (lung metastases)
  - dyspnoea (lung metastases).

Investigations
Measurement of two important serum markers – alpha-fetoprotein (αFP) and beta-human chorionic gonadotrophin (β-HCG) – should be performed before surgery and regularly during treatment and follow-up. About 90% of patients with teratoma will have either αFP or β-HCG elevated and nearly half will have both markers raised. β-HCG may be elevated in seminoma, but αFP elevation always indicates the presence of teratomatous elements. Patients are staged clinically by whole body CT scan. The staging system most commonly used in the UK is the Royal Marsden system: stage 1 (confined to testis), stage 2 (lymph nodes below the diaphragm involved), stage 3 (lymph nodes above the diaphragm involved), and stage 4 (extralymphatic disease).

Treatment
Surgery (orchidectomy through an inguinal incision) is the initial definitive treatment for all testicular tumours. Treatment thereafter depends on the histology and stage. In seminoma adjuvant radiotherapy to the ipsilateral and para-aortic lymph nodes is often recommended, though other authorities simply keep a careful follow-up on these patients with CT scans and tumour marker estimations. Likewise, in stage 1 teratoma close surveillance is the usual recom-

mended policy. Patients with more extensive disease require chemotherapy. The standard treatment for teratoma is a combination of bleomycin, etoposide and cisplatin, though high-risk patients may require more intensive regimens. In advanced seminoma, chemotherapy is given to all patients with the exception of those with minimal stage 2 disease, who are treated effectively with radiotherapy alone.

Occasionally surgery may be required for residual masses.

Prognosis

Overall the prognosis of testicular tumours is excellent, even in patients with advanced disease. For patients with stage 1 disease, cure can be expected in over 90% of cases, while even with more advanced stages over three-quarters are cured. Relapse is most common in the first 12–18 months but occasionally late relapses are seen and the risk of second tumours should not be overlooked.

Prostate

Basic facts

Carcinoma of the prostate is a disease primarily of elderly men. Its incidence is increasing and it is a common coincidental post-mortem finding in men dying over the age of 85. It is rare below the age of 45. The main aetiological factors are:

- genetic susceptibility in young patients

- (benign prostatic hyperplasia).

Pathology

Prostate tumours are typically adenocarcinomas and develop most frequently in the peripheral parts of the gland, often multifocally. Tumours may be graded histologically to give prognostic information and positive staining is usually seen for acid phosphatase and prostate-specific antigen (PSA). The tumour spreads both by local infiltration into surrounding tissues and via the bloodstream, particularly through the vertebral plexus of veins to the skeleton. Lymph node and other blood-borne metastases are uncommon.

Clinical features

Symptoms and signs therefore arise from:

- the primary tumour itself
  – bone pain
  – spinal cord compression.

- bloodstream spread
  – bone pain
  – spinal cord compression.

Investigations
Histological diagnosis is usually confirmed by transurethral resection of the prostate or by needle biopsy through the rectal mucosa. Bone metastases may be identified by X-ray and/or isotope bone scan, and imaging of the pelvis by ultrasound or CT will give information on the extent of the tumour. The tumour is usually staged A to D (A, coincidental finding; B, locally confined; C, locally advanced; and D, metastases).

Treatment
For patients with localized disease the choice is between surgery (radical prostatectomy) and radiotherapy. For patients with metastatic disease, responses may be seen with hormone therapy (surgical orchidectomy, oestrogens, anti-androgens and gonadotrophin-releasing hormone agonists).

Chemotherapy is rarely effective; for bone metastases radiotherapy, bone-seeking radioisotopes and bisphosphonates may be of palliative value.

Prognosis
Survival is best in localized disease treated radically; over three-quarters of such patients live longer than five years. Although the natural history of prostate cancer may be indolent, with locally or systemically advanced disease five-year survival falls to below 50% and 20%, respectively.

Urinary tract

Bladder

Basic facts
Malignant tumours of the bladder generally affect elderly men in their 70s and 80s. Around 10 000 cases are seen in the UK each year. They rarely present before the age of 50 and affect twice as many men as women. The main aetiological factors are:

- chemical carcinogens

- smoking

- chronic irritation (diverticuli, calculi, schistosomiasis).

Pathology
Bladder cancers usually develop as papillomas which if untreated will progress to invasive carcinoma. They are often multiple and may vary histologically through all grades, from well differentiated to poorly differentiated anaplastic tumours. In the UK more than 90% are transitional cell carcinomas, most frequently affecting the base and lateral walls of the bladder and then invading locally into muscle and then perivesical fat. Spread is via the lymph nodes in the pelvis and para-aortic region, and via the bloodstream, particularly to the lungs and bone.

Clinical features
Symptoms and signs therefore arise from:

- the primary tumour itself
  –painless haematuria
  –other urinary symptoms (frequency, urgency dysuria)

- metastatic spread
  –uncommon.

Investigations
Bladder cancer is usually staged using the TNM (tumour, node, metastasis) staging system, the extent of the tumour being the most important feature. Diagnosis is usually from biopsy taken at the time of cystoscopy, though cytological examination of the urine may reveal malignant cells. CT scan may be necessary to delineate the extent of the tumour.

Treatment
Small superficial well differentiated tumours, whether single or multiple, are best treated by transurethral resection followed by careful and frequent repeat cystoscopic examination, to treat recurrences (which occur in over half of patients). Intravesical chemotherapy is also useful for controlling superficial bladder cancer. For progressive disease the choice is between radiotherapy and surgery, each of which has its own side effects. In many centres cystectomy, with or without additional radiotherapy, is the preferred treatment. For those too

frail to tolerate radical treatment, palliative radiotherapy will dramatically relieve symptoms. The role of systemic chemotherapy in routine management has yet to be defined.

Prognosis
The prognosis of bladder cancer is very dependent on the extent of the tumour – ranging from 70% long-term survival for superficial carcinomas down to less than 10% where there has been extravesical spread.

Kidney

Basic facts
Renal cell carcinoma (hypernephroma) is the usual malignant tumour of the kidney in adults, with males affected slightly more frequently than females. It arises most commonly in the sixth and seventh decades of life. The main aetiological factor is smoking.

Pathology
These tumours are adenocarcinomas composed of cells with characteristically clear cytoplasm showing variable differentiation. Local extension of the tumour into the renal vein and then into the inferior vena cava is common. The tumour invades the surrounding kidney and may spread via the lymph nodes to the renal hilar and para-aortic nodes or via the bloodstream, particularly to lung and bone.

Clinical features
Symptoms and signs therefore arise from:

* the primary tumour itself
  – haematuria
  – loin pain
  – palpable loin mass

* local extension of the primary tumour
  – back pain

* bloodstream spread
  – pathological fracture (bone involvement)
  – dyspnoea (lung involvement)

- paraneoplastic syndromes
  - fever
  - polycythaemia (erythropoietin overproduction).

Investigations

Apart from routine blood investigations the most useful test is an ultrasound scan, which often facilitates tissue diagnosis by 'guided' biopsy. A chest X-ray can be helpful in detecting lung metastases.

Treatment

Surgery is the only curative therapy and where possible radical nephrectomy should be performed. Once renal cell carcinoma has spread, management is difficult. Occasionally spontaneous regression of metastases may occur after removal of the primary tumour, and some patients show responses to progestogen therapy (e.g. medroxyprogesterone acetate).

Chemotherapy is ineffective but certain biological therapies (particularly with interferon and interleukin II) have been shown to give sustained remissions; current research studies are likely to define the true place of these expensive and sometimes toxic agents.

Occasionally renal cell cancer is associated with solitary metastasis; surgical resection of such lesions can be appropriate.

Prognosis

The prognosis of renal cell carcinoma is better when the tumour has been radically excised (over two-thirds of patients survive five years or longer). Even where metastases are present patients may have a long and indolent natural history, but few survive more than five years.

Skin

Basic facts

Skin cancer is one of the commonest human malignancies. Basal cell carcinoma accounts for over half, and squamous cell carcinomas for over a quarter of all skin cancers. The remaining proportion is made up of melanoma, secondary skin metastases, lymphoma and various other uncommon lesions. The main aetiological factors are:

- white skin

- excessive sunlight exposure

- genetic susceptibility

- chemical carcinogenesis

- chronic irritation.

Pathology

Basal cell carcinoma (rodent ulcer) arises most commonly in the head and neck region, characteristically as an ulcerated nodule. Metastases are rare and if death occurs it is usually from infiltration of vital structures, particularly the brain, where infection is often the terminal event.

Squamous cell carcinoma occurs in the head and neck region in over half of cases, and on the arms and hands in about a quarter. Bowen's disease, usually manifested as brownish-red crusted or eroded skin plaques, is a form of intraepidermal carcinoma which may become invasive after a period of months or years; it is also acknowledged to be a herald marker of internal malignancy, particularly lung cancer.

Malignant melanoma is being seen with increasing incidence. It is divided into three types: lentigo maligna (a flat dark brown lesion occurring classically on the head and neck region of the older patient), superficial spreading melanoma (flat and extending, usually nearly black in colour), and nodular melanoma (sometimes ulcerated and usually dark brown).

Treatment

The vast majority of basal cell carcinomas are cured by surgical excision or by local radiotherapy. Likewise, excisional surgery is usually successful with squamous cell carcinoma. However, larger poorly differentiated lesions may infiltrate extensively and metastasize by lymphatic and vascular invasion. Surgery may still be appropriate but radiotherapy is particularly useful in this group, and disseminated disease occasionally responds to combination cytotoxic chemotherapy.

Treatment of primary melanoma must be by adequate excisional surgery. Once metastasis has occurred prognosis is bad. For regional recurrence, block dissection of nodes or arterial limb perfusion with cytotoxic agents is occasionally effective. For widespread disease, radiotherapy may give symptomatic relief to local deposits; palliation may be seen in a small proportion of patients with metastatic disease using agents such as dacarbazine and interferon.

Prognosis

Basal cell and squamous cell carcinomas have an excellent prognosis: over 90% of these will be cured by local treatment. For melanoma, prognosis depends on the level of invasion of the skin: the deeper the spread the worse the prognosis. For shallow localized lesions, survival figures are excellent (over 90% at five years). Once lymph node metastasis has occurred, however, the outlook is much worse, with a five-year survival of less than 30%. Very few patients with metastasis via the bloodstream (lung, liver, brain) survive more than a few months.

Malignant lymphoma

Basic facts

Malignant lymphoma is divided into two groups, Hodgkin's disease and non-Hodgkin's lymphoma, which show some similarities but also many contrasting features. Though not common, the incidence of malignant lymphoma (particularly of the non-Hodgkin's type) is increasing. Non-Hodgkin's lymphoma is commoner than Hodgkin's disease (in a ratio of 3 or 4:1). Hodgkin's disease, described by Thomas Hodgkin in 1832, has a bimodal age incidence, one peak occurring at 15–34 years and the other after 50; it is commoner in males than females, particularly in the older age group. High-grade non-Hodgkin's lymphomas arise in all age groups, though their incidence increases with age, whilst low-grade tumours are commonest in later life. The main aetiological factors are:

- viruses

- genetic factors

- radiation exposure

- previous cytotoxic chemotherapy.

Pathology

The histopathological diagnosis is made by biopsy of the involved tissue, usually lymph node. In Hodgkin's disease the characteristic cell is the Reed–Sternberg cell. The Rye classification describes the histological types of Hodgkin's disease:

lymphocyte-predominant, nodular sclerosis, mixed cellularity and lymphocyte-depletion.

Classification of non-Hodgkin's lymphomas remains complicated and they are often simply referred to as low- and high-grade as broad management groups; the grading is done on the basis of morphological and immunological features.

Clinical features

Two-thirds of patients with Hodgkin's disease will present with cervical lymphadenopathy; spread of the disease is contiguous. Non-Hodgkin's lymphomas often present with more generalized lymph node disease; about 25% start in extranodal tissues, for example tonsils, gut and skin.

Investigations

Histological confirmation is mandatory, usually by lymph node or other biopsy. Staging is according to the Ann Arbor criteria, summarized as stage 1 (localized lymphadenopathy), stage 2 (regional lymphadenopathy), stage 3 (generalized lymphadenopathy) and stage 4 (generalized lymphadenopathy plus extralymphatic involvement). The patient is also then graded according to his symptom status: A (asymptomatic), and B (symptomatic, significant weight loss and/or night sweats and/or unexplained persistent fever). Unfavourable prognostic markers are older age, male sex, unfavourable histological type, widespread bulky and symptomatic disease, low haemoglobin, low lymphocyte count (in Hodgkin's disease), high erythrocyte sedimentation rate, low serum albumin, high serum lactic dehydrogenase (in high-grade non-Hodgkin's lymphoma), and poor response to initial therapy.

Treatment

Treatment must be planned on the basis of clinical, histopathological and investigative findings. Localized Hodgkin's disease is treated primarily by radical mega-voltage wide-field radiotherapy with areas adjacent to involved sites often being irradiated prophylactically – for example with the 'Mantle' technique. For advanced Hodgkin's disease cyclical chemotherapy is appropriate, for example with regimens such as MOPP (mustine, Oncovin [vincristine], procarbazine, prednisolone) and ABVD (Adriamycin, [doxorubicin], bleomycin, vinblastine, dacarbazine). Sometimes the treatments are combined (combined modality).

For non-Hodgkin's lymphoma, localized (stage 1 – nodal or extranodal) disease is potentially curable by local radical irradiation. For more widespread non-Hodgkin's lymphoma, with high-grade histology types, intensive intravenous chemotherapy is appropriate; a combination of cyclophosphamide, Hydroxydaunorubicin (doxorubicin), Oncovin and prednisolone (CHOP) is commonly used.

For low-grade non-Hodgkin's lymphoma an expectant policy may be appropriate, instituting treatment only when the patient's lymphadenopathy becomes symptomatic, or systemic symptoms develop, or a 'vital' organ is involved. This may involve local low-dose irradiation, combination chemotherapy, or more commonly single-agent oral chemotherapy (e.g. chlorambucil).

Autologous bone marrow, or peripheral blood stem cell, transplantation is a very exciting area of development which will undoubtedly improve the outlook for patients with Hodgkin's disease not responding to, or relapsing after, conventional chemotherapy. In non-Hodgkin's lymphoma its role is less clear, particularly since we are conscious that 'salvage' treatment very rarely helps after first-line conventional chemotherapy failure. The role of 'transplant' as part-and-parcel of first-line treatment protocols is therefore being evaluated.

Prognosis

In Hodgkin's disease, for localized disease there is at least an 80% chance of long-term disease-free survival; with widespread disease treated by chemotherapy, 75% complete remission is seen, and over half of these patients will be cured.

With high-grade non-Hodgkin's lymphoma, the prognosis varies enormously with histology and stage: survival rates of 60–80% disease-free at five years for localized disease and 30–40% for widespread disease are seen.

With low-grade lymphoma the median survival is 7–8 years, whatever the treatment.

Head and neck

Basic facts

Head and neck cancers account for only a small percentage of patients presenting with cancer; however, the complexity of their management results in a disproportionately high work-load. The head and neck region is a complex area with many different structures, but includes the lips, mouth, oropharynx, postnasal space, nasal cavity and paranasal sinuses, larynx, salivary glands and thyroid gland. The main aetiological factors are:

- smoking (squamous carcinoma)

- alcohol (squamous carcinoma)

- wood workers (adenocarcinoma)

- chewing tobacco, betel nut leaf and slaked lime plug (Indian subcontinent)

- Epstein–Barr virus (South-East Asia).

Pathology

Malignant tumours of the larynx are the commonest head and neck cancers (other than skin tumours), followed by tumours of the mouth and oropharynx (including the tonsil) and nasopharynx. 90% of the tumours are epithelial and of squamous type. Adenocarcinomas occur in less than 5% of cases (particularly in the salivary glands and thyroid). Other tumours occur less commonly, for example sarcomas and melanomas. Involvement of lymph nodes is very common with squamous cell carcinoma of the head and neck.

Clinical features

Symptoms and signs therefore arise from:

- the primary tumour itself
  - symptomatic lump
  - hoarseness (laryngeal carcinoma)
  - nasal obstruction/discharge/bleeding (nasopharyngeal tumour)
  - deafness (nasopharyngeal tumour)

- local extension of the primary tumour
  - cranial nerve lesions (nasopharyngeal tumour)

- lymphatic spread to regional nodes
  - cervical lymphadenopathy

- bloodstream spread
  - bone/lung lesions (follicular carcinoma of the thyroid)

- paraneoplastic syndromes
  - systemic (anorexia, cachexia)
  - endocrine (hypercalcaemia – squamous carcinomas).

Investigations

Clinical (ENT) examination is of paramount importance. MRI and CT scans are invaluable in determining the extent of disease.

Treatment

Curative treatment for head and neck cancer involves the choice of surgery, radiotherapy, or a combination of these; the choice should be determined following preliminary discussions between surgeon and oncologist. Supportive care is very important (particularly nutritional support).

Chemotherapy may have a role in palliation (using drugs such as cisplatin).

For well differentiated (follicular and papillary) thyroid carcinomas, residual tumour activity may be ablated by administration of iodine-131.

Prognosis

Early tumours fare well, with above 70% five-year survival. Once lymphatic spread has occurred the survival falls to below 25%. Survival obviously depends on the primary site of the cancer, being best in laryngeal carcinoma and worst in nasopharyngeal tumours.

Central nervous system

Basic facts

Primary tumours of the CNS are uncommon, accounting for less than 2% of all tumours. They can arise at all ages, with two age peaks – one in childhood and the other in later life. About two-thirds of paediatric CNS tumours are infratentorial and a similar proportion in adults are supratentorial. Overall there is no difference in sex incidence. The main aetiological factors are:

- genetic predisposition

- immunosuppression (lymphomas).

Pathology

Malignant tumours of the CNS are unique in that they seldom metastasize outside their system of origin; they are, however, locally invasive, and some (for example medulloblastoma) have a tendency to spread along the CSF pathways. Benign tumours can produce pressure symptoms and clinical sequelae similar to those of malignant tumours.

Gliomas comprise approximately 50–60% of all primary central nervous system tumours, astrocytomas accounting for the vast majority of these. They are graded histologically high- or low-grade. Others include oligodendroglioblastomas, ependymomas and medulloblastomas. Meningiomas are the commonest tumour of the meninges. Schwannomas arise from the nerve sheath: an example of this is the acoustic neuroma, occurring in the auditory nerve. Embryonal tumours include craniopharyngioma arising from the embryological remnant of Rathke's pouch, and chordoma. Pituitary gland tumours are usually adenomas and are capable of producing a range of hormones. Rare tumours include pineoblastoma, dysgerminoma, teratoma, haemangioma and lymphoma.

Metastatic tumours are very common in the brain and account for approximately one-fifth of all cerebral tumours.

Spinal cord tumours may develop in the extradural or intradural compartments – extradural tumours are most commonly metastatic in origin, intradural tumours include neurofibroma and meningioma (which are extramedullary) and astrocytoma and ependymoma (intramedullary).

Clinical features

Symptoms and signs therefore arise from:

* the primary tumour itself
  – raised intracranial pressure (headache, vomiting, papilloedema – later associated with reduced level of consciousness)
  – false localizing signs (e.g. VI cranial nerve palsy)
  – localized symptoms and signs (visual field defects from pituitary tumours)
  – personality change from frontal lobe tumours
  – epilepsy
  – back pain (spinal cord tumours)
  – paraplegia (spinal cord tumours).

Diagnosis

Decisions on management require precise knowledge of the extent as well as the site of the lesion, and a firm histological diagnosis. CT scan is now the investigation of choice for brain tumours. MRI may also be useful (particularly for spinal cord, brainstem and posterior fossa lesions).

Treatment

The initial management usually involves some form of surgical intervention to establish a histological diagnosis and, depending on size and location, to debulk the tumour.

Radiotherapy is useful with some tumours but radiosensitivity varies widely, with pineal dysgerminomas being highly radiosensitive and meningiomas and low-grade gliomas being radioresistant.

Chemotherapy in general has a limited role in the treatment of CNS tumours, except in certain less common tumours.

Primary spinal cord tumours are treated by surgical excision (debulking) and in most cases this is followed by postoperative radiotherapy.

Prognosis

The five-year survival of low-grade gliomas is about 50% after appropriate surgery. For high-grade gliomas, median survival is less than a year. Medulloblastoma, with treatment involving both radiotherapy and chemotherapy, has an average five-year survival rate of around 45%. Surgical resection of meningiomas and craniopharyngiomas gives excellent results. Surgery, often followed by postoperative irradiation, gives long-term control in the majority of pituitary tumours.

The treatment of cerebral metastasis is palliative in intent. High-dose steroids (usually dexamethasone) are a very useful measure in the short-term treatment of raised intracranial pressure. Depending on the primary site, palliative radiotherapy may be useful, and occasionally if the metastasis is solitary, surgical removal is appropriate.

Malignant spinal cord compression requires urgent treatment – surgery, radiotherapy and steroids are used singly or in combination. The overall prognosis for this syndrome remains very poor and is related to the pretreatment neurological status and the radioresponsiveness of the primary malignancy.

Leukaemia

Basic facts

Acute lymphoblastic leukaemia (ALL) is the commonest leukaemia in childhood and acute myeloid leukaemia (AML) is the commonest in adults. Chronic myeloid leukaemia is relatively uncommon and occurs most commonly in the 30–60-year age group. Chronic lymphocytic leukaemia is a disease of late middle age and old age. Acute leukaemia is often florid and aggressive in clinical presentation; chronic leukaemias are more indolent in their behaviour. The main aetiological factors are:

- genes (e.g. increased incidence in Down's syndrome)
- radiation
- certain chemicals (e.g. benzene)
- viruses (e.g. human T-cell lymphotrophic virus type 1).

Pathology

A number of classification systems exist (one of the commonest being the French/American/British – FAB – for acute leukaemia) which classify the blast cells by morphology.

Clinical features

Symptoms and signs may therefore arise from:

- bone marrow infiltration
  - anaemia
  - bruising/bleeding
  - infection
  - bone pain
- involvement of the lympho-reticular system
  - splenomegaly (can be massive in AML)
  - lymphadenopathy (particularly in lymphatic leukaemia)
- paraneoplastic effects
  - hyperviscosity (AML)

– coagulopathies

– systemic features (fever, malaise, weight loss).

Investigations

The diagnosis is usually made by examination of bone marrow and/or peripheral blood cells. Cytogenetic and immunocytochemical investigations are often performed. In AML the classic abnormality is a t(9; 22) translocation, the Philadelphia chromosome.

Treatment

The treatment of acute leukaemia consists of induction of remission, consolidation of remission and then either maintenance or ablative therapy. CNS prophylaxis is undertaken in ALL. Although most patients with acute leukaemia achieve remission, many relapse due to the presence of occult disease which has not been eradicated.

High-dose chemotherapy after autologous or allogenic bone marrow transplant can eradicate the occult disease. With autologous bone marrow (or peripheral stem cell) transplantation there is a very real risk of reinfusing malignant cells; bone marrow purging may be undertaken. Chronic myeloid leukaemia is usually treated with single-agent chemotherapy (busulfan or hydroxyurea). In younger patients more intensive treatments (including high-dose chemotherapy) may be effective. In chronic lymphocytic leukaemia, treatment is palliative with alkylating agents such as chlorambucil or cyclophosphamide.

Prognosis

In general the prognosis is good with a cure rate in excess of 70% in ALL, and even in AML now over 30%. Chronic myeloid leukaemia has a median survival of 3–4 years. Chronic lymphocytic leukaemia is a slowly progressive disorder with a median survival of over ten years, patients often dying of other causes.

Childhood tumours

Cancer in children is relatively rare; nevertheless, it is the third commonest cause of death in childhood. There are many different types of cancer, but approximately one-third will have leukaemia, one-third brain tumours and the other third will be composed of a variety of tumours, including Wilms' tumour, neuroblastoma, lymphomas and soft-tissue sarcomas.

The causes of childhood cancer are an area of considerable interest; genetic factors play an important part; most tumours do not have a clearly defined inheritance (with the exception of retinoblastoma, for example) but the incidence of cancer in siblings is higher than one would expect in a normal population.

In general the outlook for children with cancer has improved dramatically since the introduction of chemotherapy: at least half of these cancers are cured and for many types survival rates are much higher than they were just 30 years ago (Figure 5.1).

Particular problems for managing children include those of psychosocial and communication issues, the major problems of immunosuppression and infection, and the possibility of early metabolic upset. Childhood cancers should therefore only be treated in specialist paediatric oncology centres, mostly in the context of national studies.

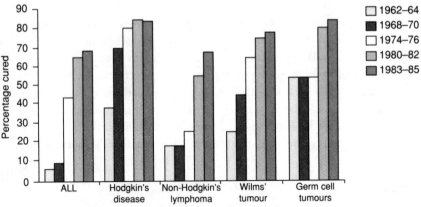

Figure 5.1:   Childhood cancer: improvements in survival.

Sarcomas

Soft-tissue sarcomas account for approximately 1% of adult cancers; they are relatively more common in children (6–7%) because of the reduced number of carcinomas in this group. There is no clear cause for the majority of cases, though there are well established associations with genetic linked disorders such as von Recklinghausen's neurofibromatosis, tuberous sclerosis, the basal cell naevus and Li–Fraumeni syndromes. Previous exposure to ionizing radiation may be a factor; it is not clear whether there is a causative relationship with trauma. Many soft-tissue sarcomas have consistent chromosome rearrangements. Histological diagnosis is essential; tumours are graded high- or low-grade, the majority falling into the high-grade category. Histological grade is important in determining prognosis; also important are tumour size, nodal involvement and the presence of metastases.

CT or MRI scans are appropriate radiological investigations. Specialized surgery is important and may involve anything from very local excision through to radical ablative surgery (for example in extremity tumours).

Adjuvant radiotherapy is of confirmed value and though the majority of adult soft tissue sarcomas are chemoresistant there is a small group of tumours for which chemotherapy is the primary treatment (using combinations including vincristine, doxorubicin, cyclophosphamide and dactinomycin).

The overall survival of patients with soft-tissue sarcoma varies from 35 to 70% depending on patient selection; in general young age, extremity tumour, small size and low-grade histology are good prognostic features.

Ewing's sarcoma usually occurs in the second decade of life; it is commoner in males, presents with pain and swelling in the affected region and in up to a third of cases is metastatic in presentation. It most commonly presents in the femur and bones of the pelvis, but may affect any bone. Treatment is usually by primary surgical resection, followed by chemotherapy and local radiotherapy. With such combinations of treatment five-year survival is now seen in about one-third of patients; this is obviously for localized disease and distal primary tumour.

Osteosarcoma is very rare, occurs during childhood and adolescence and is treated at special centres. Limb-sparing surgery with neo-adjuvant or adjuvant chemotherapy has improved the overall survival to over 60%.

Further reading

Abeloff M D, Armitage J O, Lichter A S *et al.* (eds) (1995) *Clinical Oncology,* Churchill Livingstone, New York.

De Vita V T, Hellman S and Rosenberg S A (eds) (1994) *Cancer–Principles and Practice of Oncology* (4th edn), J B Lippincott, Philadelphia, USA.

Peckham M (joint ed.) (1995) *Oxford Textbook of Oncology,* Oxford Medical Publications, Oxford.

Souhami R and Tobias J (1995) *Cancer and its Management* (2nd edn), Blackwell Science Ltd, Oxford.

6

Oncological emergencies

R E Coleman

Introduction

The management of cancer generally follows a well ordered path of diagnosis, staging and treatment. However, at some stage in the disease many patients will experience a sudden severe upset caused by the disease or treatment: a so-called oncological emergency. The more common conditions are listed in Table 6.1. An understanding of these conditions is important to all health-care professionals encountering cancer patients as, in addition to causing unpleasant symptoms, they may result in permanent disability or even death if not treated or recognized promptly.

Infection (particularly if neutropenic)
Haemorrhage
Hypercalcaemia of malignancy
Spinal cord compression
Pathological fractures
Superior vena cava obstruction
Pericardial tamponade
Bowel obstruction
Seizures

Table 6.1: Common oncological emergencies

Infection

Cancer patients are particularly susceptible to infection. Cellular and humoral immunity may be impaired by the disease, and specific organ damage may predispose to the entry of pathogens. In addition, many patients are both malnourished and immobile and may have venous or urinary catheters in situ.

However, it is the additional myelosuppressive effect of treatment, particularly chemotherapy, which increases the risk of infection the most. For many chemotherapy regimens neutropenia is greatest 7–14 days after administration, and it is during this nadir of the white cell count that infection is most likely. The probability of infection during myelosuppression is related to both the absolute level and duration of neutropenia, with the probability of infection rising to above 50% in those experiencing neutropenia of less than $0.5 \times 10^9/L$ for more than five days.

The patient may present in a variety of ways. Fever and specific signs of infection may be present but are not invariable. Often the patient suddenly becomes generally unwell, perhaps appearing confused or drowsy. All patients possibly suffering from neutropenic sepsis should be assessed immediately. In just a few hours an untreated episode of neutropenic sepsis may progress to become overwhelming, with septic shock, renal failure and death.

Patients becoming unwell at home should be visited urgently by their GP. Often urgent admission to hospital is the best policy, but if the patient appears reasonably well and it is possible to visit again within a few hours to check on progress, patients may stay at home on an oral broad-spectrum antibiotic. A blood sample should always be taken for an urgent blood count. If a blood count result cannot be guaranteed within a few hours or the patient cannot be reassessed by the same doctor, then immediate admission to hospital is recommended.

On arrival in the hospital a blood count and blood culture should be performed. If neutropenia is confirmed, broad-spectrum intravenous antibiotics should be commenced without delay. Most hospitals have an antibiotic policy for febrile neutropenia, and a number of these are listed in Table 6.2. Additional investigations include urine microscopy and culture, a chest radiograph, swabs and cultures from central venous catheter lines and sputum culture. Often the patient's symptoms or signs will dictate which investigations are the most important.

Intravenous antibiotics should continue until the patient has been apyrexial for at least 24–48 hours, after which oral therapy should be given for 5–7

Ciprofloxacin +/- flucloxacillin or vancomycin
Ceftazidime +/- flucloxacillin or vancomycin
Piperacillin + gentamicin or amikacin

Table 6.2: Common antibiotic regimens for neutropenic fever

days. Bacteriological confirmation of septicaemia is obtained in only 20–30% of cases of neutropenic fever. However, positive cultures when isolated are very helpful in confirming the choice of antibiotic and directing the selection of oral follow-on therapy.

In patients with profound neutropenia it may be necessary to continue intravenous antibiotics. If fever continues, consideration should be given to adding antimicrobial agents for viral infection (particularly for herpes simplex), fungal sepsis (particularly candida) and protozoal infections (*Pneumocystis carinii*). Fungal and protozoal infections are much more of a problem in patients with prolonged severe neutropenia caused by treatment of leukaemia or following bone marrow transplantation. In the context of solid tumour oncology they are relatively rare.

Haemorrhage

Bleeding problems are very common in cancer patients. Haemorrhage may occur from the tumour, particularly from those arising in the gastrointestinal tract. Peptic ulceration is also frequent, often induced by drugs such as nonsteroidal anti-inflammatory agents or corticosteroids and exacerbated by stress and poor nutrition. Clotting may also be defective, as a result of either liver dysfunction or bone marrow infiltration, or more frequently secondary to cytotoxic drug treatment.

Patients with significant blood loss or at risk of major haemorrhage require admission for haematological support and, where possible, treatment of the underlying cause. Red cell transfusions are required for anaemia and platelet transfusion should be considered in patients with severe thrombocytopenia, particularly if they are actively bleeding. The threshold for transfusing platelets is disputed but the risk of cerebral haemorrhage increases rapidly when the platelet count falls below $10 \times 10^9/L$, and a platelet transfusion may be lifesaving in patients with active bleeding associated with thrombocytopenia. Clotting abnormalities are best corrected by infusion of fresh frozen plasma.

Anti-ulcer drugs, including the H_2 antagonists cimetidine and ranitidine, and the newer proton pump inhibitors and prostaglandin analogues are all helpful in the prevention and treatment of idiopathic or drug-induced peptic ulceration. Occasionally surgical intervention, endoscopic techniques for achieving haemostasis and interventional radiological techniques of embolization will be needed for intractable or life-threatening haemorrhage.

Hypercalcaemia of malignancy

Hypercalcaemia is the commonest metabolic complication of malignancy. It may develop as a result of widespread bone destruction by metastases or secondary to the humoral effects of bone-resorbing factors, particularly parathyroid hormone-related peptide (PTHrP) released by the tumour. Hypercalcaemia is most common in breast cancer and multiple myeloma, where local osteolytic bone destruction predominates, and in squamous tumours of the bronchus or head and neck, when humoral mechanisms are more frequent.

Hypercalcaemia causes a number of symptoms and signs (see Table 6.3), the severity of which are related to the height of the serum calcium and the speed with which hypercalcaemia has developed. Dehydration is inevitable as calcium is a potent diuretic, but many of the symptoms are non-specific and easily confused with more general features of the malignancy and its treatment.

Once hypercalcaemia of malignancy has developed it is unlikely to resolve without specific treatment and referral to hospital is usually required. The treatment of choice is rehydration, initially with intravenous normal saline, plus inhibition of osteoclast-mediated bone destruction with a biphosphonate such as pamidronate or clodronate. Treatment will restore normocalcaemia in 70–100% of patients within 3–5 days.

Where possible acute control of hypercalcaemia should be followed by appropriate anti-cancer treatment to control the underlying malignancy. This is usually chemotherapy or endocrine therapy as metastases are generally present,

---

Nausea and vomiting
Polyuria and polydipsia
Dehydration
Malaise and weakness
Constipation
Bone pain
Confusion
Drowsiness
Dysarthria
Hyporeflexia
Convulsions
Cardiac dysrhythmias

Table 6.3: Symptoms and signs of hypercalcaemia

but in the case of a primary lung or head and neck tumour local radiotherapy may be effective. When this is not possible hypercalcaemia is likely to recur as the effects of the bisphosphonate wane. Repeated intravenous administration of pamidronate every 3–4 weeks, or possibly oral clodronate therapy, may continue to provide useful palliation. The average survival after an episode of hypercalcaemia is three months.

In general, despite the poor prognosis, hypercalcaemia is a worthwhile complication of malignancy to treat, leading to symptomatic improvement and a better quality of life for the patient. However, occasionally treatment is not appropriate and the condition is best allowed to progress as a terminal event.

Spinal cord compression

This is a devastating complication of advanced malignancy usually occurring in patients with metastatic bone disease. Damage to the spinal cord may be due to fracture dislocation of damaged vertebrae or soft-tissue extension of metastases into the epidural space. Typically patients complain of weakness with or without numbness of the legs, often associated with pain in the back and a past history of metastatic bone disease.

Rapid diagnosis, assessment and treatment are essential if neurological damage is not to become permanent. Patients should be admitted and assessed in detail. Neurological examination may reveal a sensory level above which the compression must lie. Plain radiographs may show obvious bony destruction, but usually additional imaging tests are required. MRI is the investigation of choice as it allows assessment of the entire spine without the hazards or discomfort of myelography. Multiple sites of compression may be revealed. However, when MRI is not available a lumbar myelogram is recommended. If this shows a complete block a cervical myelogram may also be necessary to delineate the top of the obstruction and any more proximal levels of compression. CT scanning of the site of compression may also give useful structural information.

All patients should be started on high-dose corticosteroids to reduce oedema around the site of compression while a decision on definitive treatment is made. The choice between radiotherapy and surgical management of cord compression depends on many factors, including the nature of the underlying disease, general fitness and prognosis of the patient, and the severity of the neurological damage. In general, surgical decompression is only performed for those reasonably fit patients with rapidly progressive neurology of recent onset

(< 24 hours), or where the diagnosis is either unknown so that a tissue diagnosis can be made or is known to respond relatively poorly to radiotherapy treatment. All other patients are usually treated with radiotherapy, but a few with lymphoma or small-cell lung cancer may also benefit from concomitant chemotherapy.

The prognosis for spinal cord compression is profoundly influenced by the severity of neurological dysfunction before treatment. Those patients diagnosed early and in whom treatment can be started before complete paralysis and sphincter control have developed have a much better chance of neurological recovery. Patients with complete paralysis of more than 48 hours do not recover: radiotherapy in this situation may relieve any accompanying back pain but cannot be expected to reverse the neurological damage.

Corticosteroids, while invaluable in acute control of spinal cord compression, should be reduced as soon as possible to prevent steroid myopathy, unsightly weight gain, gastrointestinal problems and further immunosuppression.

Pathological fracture

Bone metastases typically cause progressive bone destruction and this may result in fracture. Vertebral collapse and rib fractures are the most common, and may cause pain, kyphoscoliosis and a degree of restrictive lung disease. However, it is fracture of a long bone which causes most disability. Because the development of a fracture is so devastating to a cancer patient, increasing emphasis is being placed on attempts to predict metastases at risk of fracture and the use of pre-emptive surgery.

Fractures are common through lytic metastases and weight-bearing bones, the proximal femora being the most commonly affected sites. Damage to both trabecular and cortical bone is structurally important but it is the relevance of cortical destruction which is most clearly appreciated. Over the years several radiological features have been identified which may predict imminent fracture. Fracture is likely if lesions are large (> 2 cm), are predominantly lytic and erode the cortex. Prophylactic internal fixation is the treatment of choice for such lesions, followed by radiotherapy. It is easier to stabilize a bone while it is still intact. This avoids unpleasant pain and complications for the patient, and rehabilitation and convalescence are much shorter and easier. If the patient is not fit for surgery then radiotherapy and non-weight-bearing is indicated.

Untreated pathological fractures rarely heal and although radiotherapy may achieve local tumour control, bony union remains unlikely. Radiotherapy inhibits chondrogenesis, a prerequisite for fracture healing, and with large areas of bone destruction there may be insufficient matrix remaining for adequate repair. Once a pathological fracture has occurred internal fixation is the only treatment modality likely to restore function. Prior to surgery, a radionuclide bone scan and radiographs of the entire length of the affected bone should be obtained. This ensures that any other metastases which may subsequently fracture are also stabilized and included in the radiotherapy field.

Superior vena cava (SVC) obstruction

Malignancy is the most common cause of obstruction to the SVC vessels either directly due to extrinsic pressure from the tumour, or secondary to thrombosis, which is also an increasingly common complication of the widespread use of long-term central venous catheters in cancer patients. Carcinoma of the bronchus is the commonest underlying malignancy but breast cancer and lymphomas are other frequent causes.

Typically the patient notices swelling and fullness in the neck, usually with facial and arm oedema, and a sense of constriction around the chest made worse by bending forward. Headache and blurring of vision may also be reported. As the condition progresses the patient is confined to sitting upright in a chair and becomes increasingly breathless.

Examination usually reveals the typical swollen facial appearance of SVC obstruction and the development of collateral vessels over the upper chest. Jugular venous pressure is markedly elevated, with loss of the normal venous wave form, respiratory stridor may be audible and papilloedema is a sign of severe and often long-standing obstruction.

Immediate management includes oxygen and nursing the patient in an upright position plus high-dose corticosteroids (dexamethasone 12–16 mg/day). Radiotherapy is generally the treatment of choice and will usually provide symptomatic relief. The dose and fractionation of treatment will depend on the underlying tumour but typically 20–30 Gy are administered over 5–10 fractions. Improvement is generally seen within the first few days of treatment. For those patients with lymphoma or small-cell lung cancer, combination chemotherapy should be given with or sometimes instead of radiotherapy, response in these chemosensitive tumours being at least as rapid as that seen after radiotherapy.

Recently, radiological stenting of the SVC has become possible and provides both a valuable alternative to radiotherapy and a second modality of treatment for those failing to respond or recurring after radiotherapy. A catheter is inserted into the SVC either from above (via the cephalic and subclavian veins) or from below (via a femoral vein). A coiled metallic mesh is then inserted along the catheter into a position where it bridges the site of obstruction. The stent is then released into the SVC where it springs open and splints the vessel, dramatically improving flow rate through it. Temporary anticoagulation is needed but after a few days the stent becomes covered in vascular endothelium and anticoagulation can be stopped. At present the use of SVC stents is restricted to specialist centres and limited by availability of vascular radiology facilities and the considerable costs of the procedure.

Pericardial tamponade

A malignant pericardial effusion is a relatively uncommon complication of malignancy. When it does develop, carcinoma of the bronchus and breast are the most frequent underlying tumours. The patient generally presents with a feeling of fullness in the chest, sometimes associated with pain and breathlessness which is made worse by lying flat. As the effusion increases in size the function of the right ventricle progressively declines, resulting in symptoms and signs of right heart failure. Examination may reveal a pulsus paradoxus, with more than 15 mm of paradox indicating significant tamponade. Typically the apex beat is difficult to palpate and the jugular venous pressure is raised, with disturbance of the normal wave form. A chest radiograph may reveal an enlarged cardiac shadow, typically referred to as a globular heart, while cardiac ultrasound is the investigation of choice to delineate the extent of the effusion and guide placement of the drainage catheter.

Drainage of the pericardial effusion provides rapid relief of the symptoms. Traditionally this was performed at the bedside via a pericardiocentesis needle with ECG monitoring. However, it is considerably safer to insert a soft pigtail catheter into the pericardial space, under ultrasound guidance, through which the fluid can drain over 24–48 hours.

Where possible, appropriate systemic treatment should be administered to control the underlying tumour. Although opinions differ, there is little good evidence to support the routine instillation of drugs into the pericardial cavity to try and prevent accumulation of pericardial fluid. If patients develop troublesome recurrence of the pericardial effusion, a formal cardiothoracic drainage procedure creating a window through which fluid can drain from the pericardial space to the pleural cavity is preferred. Radiotherapy treatment to the heart for pericardial effusions is no longer recommended.

Bowel obstruction

Carcinomas arising from the large bowel or ovary are the most common causes of bowel obstruction. The patient usually experiences abdominal distension, constipation and varying degrees of pain and vomiting. The situation is often exacerbated by opiate, induced constipation.

Surgery is the treatment of choice for a primary bowel tumour but in patients with metastatic disease conservative management is generally preferred. This involves adequate analgesia, intravenous hydration, nothing to eat or drink and nasogastric suction. Decompression and resting of the bowel will often lead to partial relief of the obstruction. For more resistant cases symptom relief may be provided by a subcutaneous infusion of diamorphine for pain, cyclizine or haloperidol for vomiting and dexamethasone to reduce oedema around the site of obstruction. Occasionally palliative surgery to relieve and/or bypass the obstruction may be indicated. Unfortunately there are often multiple sites of obstruction, with the small and large bowel being matted together by omental and peritoneal disease, and effective surgery in this situation is technically impossible.

Seizures

Convulsions may be either due to metastatic involvement of the brain and meninges or secondary to various metabolic disturbances, including hypercalcaemia, uraemia and inappropriate ADH secretion.

Irrespective of the cause, rapid control of the seizures with diazepam or similar and anticonvulsant medication are essential. Diazepam may be given by either the intravenous or rectal routes. The importance of giving a loading dose of an anticonvulsant such as phenytoin should be remembered to ensure therapeutic levels are attained rapidly. For cerebral metastases, dexamethasone will reduce symptoms and radiotherapy may be indicated. Metabolic causes should be treated in their own right.

Conclusions

Many of the complications of cancer referred to here as oncological emergencies only become so because of a delay in diagnosis and institution of appropriate treatment. A high index of suspicion and ready access to specialist cancer facilities are required to identify these problems at a stage when effective treatment is still possible and before unpleasant sequelae have developed.

Further reading

Abeloff M D, Armitage J O, Lichter A S *et al.* (eds) (1995) *Clinical Oncology*, Churchill Livingstone, New York.

De Vita V T, Hellman S and Rosenberg S A (eds) (1994) *Cancer – Principles and Practice of Oncology* (4th edn), J B Lippincott, Philadelphia, USA.

7

Palliative care

D J Brooks and S Ahmedzai

Introduction

The majority of adult patients who are diagnosed with cancer will eventually die of that cancer. Palliative care should therefore play an important part in the care of most cancer patients, and much of this care can be delivered in the community.

There is widespread confusion amongst both the public and health-care professionals about exactly what palliative care is, and how it relates to cancer and hospice services.

This chapter will define palliative care and describe the place of 'specialist' palliative care. It will also describe some of the principles of practising palliative care, with special emphasis on symptom control.

Terminology

The phrase 'terminal care' is now mostly used to refer to care of patients in their last few days or hours of life, and therefore it has unhelpfully negative connotations for patients in the earlier stages of incurable disease. It also focuses on dying and the impending death rather than the opportunities in the life that precedes death.

Similarly, as pointed out by Dame Cicely Saunders – who has been crucially influential in the development of the modern hospice movement – the words 'terminal patient' should rarely if ever be used. They give an impersonal and negative impression and the whole message of the hospice movement has been one of the unique and often creative possibilities that occur, even at the ending of life.

The first hospice was opened in the second half of the fourth century by Fabiola, a Roman matron and disciple of St Jerome, originally as a resting place for pilgrims and travellers on long journeys. Gradually they became places where the sick could be cared for in both body and spirit. These hospices lasted until the Reformation. They were not specifically for the dying, but the name was adopted for this use by Mme Jeanne Garnier in Lyons in 1842 and later used by the Sisters of Charity in founding Our Lady's Hospice in Dublin in 1879. Several hospices took their lead from these, turning the aim of the original hospices into a metaphor – caring for the bodies and souls of those travellers on a very important personal journey, on the road to death.

In the past 30 years, with the advent of St Christopher's Hospice in London, St Luke's Hospice in Sheffield and the many other hospices that followed in their wake, the emphasis has moved from predominantly nursing care to a more multidisciplinary approach which includes doctors, social workers, chaplains and other professions allied to medicine.

Many patients still think of a hospice as a place where they may be sent to die. They – like some of their professional carers – are unaware that 35% of patients are discharged from inpatient hospice care. They would often not know about day care or outpatient hospice care, or about hospice care provided in general hospitals. Hospice is, ultimately, not just bricks and mortar – it is more of a conceptual approach to care.

Against this background, the term 'palliative care' has been gaining increasing acceptance, especially in Canada and other countries in Europe where 'hospice' has inappropriate connotations of geriatric or social care. The word palliative comes from the Latin 'pallium', meaning a soldier's cloak. Palliation thus throws a cloak over the disease, without attempting to remove it. The metaphor can be extended to describe how palliative care is one piece of the armour which helps to shield a patient, and to provide a better quality of life alongside the use of surgery and oncology, which attempt to prolong it.

The use of the newer term palliative care has also emphasized the extension of care for cancer patients from the inpatient (hospice) setting for the later stages of disease to intervention at earlier stages in hospital and in the community. Furthermore, it is associated with a move towards involvement with patients suffering from diseases other than cancer.

A useful definition of palliative care has been proposed by the World Health Organization[1].

Palliative care is the active total care of patients whose disease is not responsive to curative treatment. Control of pain, of other symptoms and of psychological, social and spiritual problems, is paramount. The goal of palliative care is the achievement of the best quality of life for patients and their families. Many aspects of palliative care are also applicable earlier in the course of the illness in conjunction with anticancer treatment.

This definition reminds us that palliative care should be seen as an active form of care and that patients should never be told that 'there is nothing we can do'. Since many patients with cancer are being treated with curative intent, even though the likelihood of cure being achieved is not great, the definition should help to prevent such patients from being denied the benefits of good palliative care.

It also reminds us that while symptom control is paramount it is always in the context of an holistic approach to the care of the patient. The area of spiritual issues is not confined just to consideration of the religious needs (which are admittedly of increasing relevance in our multi-ethnic society). It extends to existential issues and questions of meaning and purpose in suffering ('Why me?', 'Why now?' etc.) which, if unaddressed, can aggravate the pain and other symptoms. The aim of palliative care – according to the World Health Organization – should always be to produce the best balance between quality of life and length of life for each individual patient, by:

- affirming life and regarding dying as a normal process

- neither hastening nor postponing death

- providing relief from pain and other distressing symptoms

- integrating the psychological and spiritual aspects of care

- offering a support system to help patients live as actively as possible until death

- offering a support system to help the family cope during the patient's illness and in their own bereavement.

Influenced no doubt by the fact that Dame Cicely Saunders first trained as a nurse then as a medical social worker before completing medical training, palliative care has always placed an emphasis on multidisciplinary care provision. The team approach to assessment and decision-making also extends to involvement of the patient and family members in the decision-making process. There is a high regard to patient autonomy and empowering the patient, who is often becoming more dependent in many other aspects of life. While the autonomy of the individual must be taken into account when sharing information with family members, the final outcome of any palliative care episode is the consequence of the experience on close family and friends. The effect on them, both in their bereavement and on how they face other life experiences, especially future illness, will last long after the patient has died.

Pain and symptom management

Whilst palliative care goes beyond symptom control, attention to detail in management of pain and other symptoms is essential to afford the patient time and space to address deeper issues. Psychosocial aspects and communication in cancer care are dealt with elsewhere in this volume and so the rest of this chapter will focus on physical symptoms.

The importance of assessment

The first principle of good symptom management is careful assessment of the whole patient. A detailed history of each symptom should be taken, remembering that what at first seems like one symptom may actually be several; patients with cancer pain have an average of four different pains, each of which may need a different approach. The history of the symptoms should include the patient's assessment of the cause and provoking factors of each symptom which, as well as aiding diagnosis, will give an understanding of the meaning a patient ascribes to the symptom. Asking the patient to relate the story of the illness from a personal point of view gives invaluable information with a particular emphasis on what has been tried before and the effect of each therapy, thus preventing repetition of previously unsuccessful approaches. (It is important, however, to be aware that some – particularly elderly – patients may misidentify previous symptom control efforts and can confuse drugs and their effects.)

The history from the patient should be supplemented by a careful perusal of all available medical and nursing notes for objective evidence of the extent of disease activity and spread, the anti-cancer therapies used to date and the effectiveness of therapeutic interventions thus far. Careful medical examination and appropriate investigations will yield further information.

In evaluating symptoms in patients with cancer it is relevant to bear in mind that the possible causes include not only the cancer itself but the oncological and even palliative treatments, the result of general debility, or concurrent disorders. In elderly patients, the effects of comorbidity can often overshadow the malignant process. Finally, the cancer can cause symptoms not only by direct local actions, but also indirectly through systemic effects such as hypercalcaemia or anaemia.

Sharing information

Fear of the unknown, especially in the face of frightening symptoms such as dyspnoea or bleeding, can have severe consequences on the patient's well-being. Explanation of possible causes and treatments can often relieve anxiety and uncertainty and in doing so provide considerable relief of symptoms by itself – paradoxically, even if the explanation confirms the patient's worst fear. Sharing information about the possible investigation and management strategies enables the patient to make a valuable contribution to the decision-making process and helps to individualize the care plan. Clearly some patients wish to devolve all decision-making responsibilities to the health-care professionals and will find being given options confusing and worrying, and so for those patients the information will have to be tailored to their needs. Family members also need information, but the patient's first rights to that knowledge should always be respected.

It is also often helpful to share realistic goals of therapy and the time-scale over which they are likely to be achieved: for instance in the case of a new pain the goals might be to have a pain-free night's sleep within 24 hours, to be pain-free at rest within 72 hours, and to be comfortable on movement (but not necessarily entirely pain-free) by 7 days.

Having set the goals it is important to monitor how they are being achieved and to reassure the patient that if they are not being achieved then there are other plans of action which will be triggered. It is best to forewarn about possible adverse reactions to therapies and to advise the patient and carers what to do if they occur. We see many patients who declare (perhaps having even been told this by another professional) that they 'cannot tolerate morphine', because the first time they took it they were sick. If they had been warned about possible nausea and provided with anti-emetics to take *if* it occurred, and also reassured that this reaction usually lasts for only a few days, then it is more likely that their pain could have been successfully controlled at their first attempt with morphine.

Many symptom problems are caused or aggravated by side effects of other therapies. This underlines the importance of reviewing whether those therapies are still necessary, even before side effects occur. Corticosteroids are particularly notorious in this regard for being given long after their effectiveness has diminished or often simply being continued when they had no benefit in the first instance.

Finally, before discussing specific symptom problems, it is important to consider drug interactions: not only those that cause toxicity but also those that just make therapeutic nonsense (e.g. a stimulant laxative and an antispasmodic).

Pain

The essential first step in good pain management is diagnosing the cause of the pain. It is inexcusable to say a patient has pain 'because of cancer'. The mechanism by which the cancer is causing the pain will be the best guide as to the ideal choice of first-line therapy.

Treat the cause

A crucial question to ask is: 'Is it possible to eradicate the cause of the pain?' For example, is there a pathological fracture which it would be appropriate to ask the orthopaedic surgeon to immobilize, or a bone metastasis where palliative radiotherapy may not only relieve the pain but reduce the risk of future fracture? Another example is constipation which is causing severe abdominal colic or aching pains: these will be best relieved once the constipation itself has been cleared. However, it will often still be necessary to give symptomatic analgesia while the other therapies are having effect.

The WHO analgesic ladder

The World Health Organization's analgesic ladder provides a useful framework to describe the stepwise approach to the use of drugs in the management of common cancer pains (Figure 7.1). For mild pains non-opioids such as paracetamol or non-steroidal anti-inflammatory drugs (NSAIDs) are the first-line treatment of choice (step 1).

In those cases where the pain is neuropathic in origin – a pain usually characterized by a throbbing, burning or tingling character sometimes associated with hypersensitivity – the addition of an 'adjuvant' drug such as an antidepressant or an anticonvulsant may be helpful.

In step 2, for a moderately severe pain or one that is no longer responding to non-opioids (perhaps with an adjuvant) the addition of a weak opioid is indicated, e.g. codeine or dihydrocodeine. Often this can be given in the form of a combination non-opioid/weak opioid preparation such as coproxamol.

Strong opioids such as morphine or fentanyl in doses titrated to the patient's requirement (in conjunction again with appropriate use of non-opioids and adjuvants) form step 3 on the WHO analgesic ladder. (Occasionally step 2 is omitted in favour of starting a patient previously on a non-opioid or NSAID only directly onto a small dose of strong opioid.) Whichever formulation or route of administration is chosen as most appropriate for the patient it is essential that the frequency of dosing is adequate to maintain serum levels in the therapeutic range. For instance, with oral instant-release liquid or tablet morphine, this means regular four-hourly administration; with sustained-release

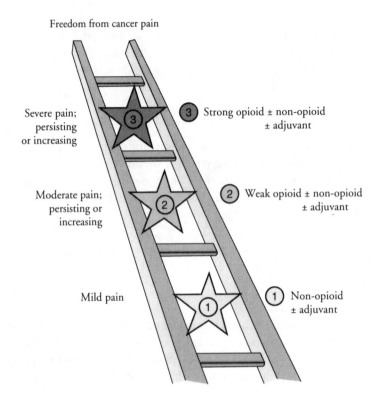

Freedom from cancer pain

Severe pain; persisting or increasing — ③ Strong opioid ± non-opioid ± adjuvant

Moderate pain; persisting or increasing — ② Weak opioid ± non-opioid ± adjuvant

Mild pain — ① Non-opioid ± adjuvant

Figure 7.1:   The World Health Organization's 'analgesic ladder' (adapted from World Health Organization, 1990).

formulations it means 12-hourly dosing. The new transdermal fentanyl patch can be changed every three days.

Local interventions such as transcutaneous electrical nerve stimulation (TENS), nerve blocks, epidural or intrathecal injections or infusions may be helpful in selected patients under specialist supervision, e.g. from a hospice or hospital specialist team, or from a pain clinic.

Common gastrointestinal symptoms

Constipation

Constipation is a frequent and troublesome symptom. The cause is often drug-related. Opioids inhibit forward peristalsis to varying degrees and drugs with anticholinergic activity (e.g. tricyclic antidepressants, hyoscine, cyclizine and methotrimeprazine) reduce all bowel contractions. However, other causes such as immobility, anorexia, dehydration, intra-abdominal malignancy, denervation and hypercalcaemia are also common causes. Intestinal obstruction should always be excluded as a possible cause of constipation as this will require a different approach.

Some of these causes are clearly reversible, e.g. hypercalcaemia, which may be treated with intravenous bisphosphonates with dramatic effect. Others may be predicted, e.g. opioid-related constipation, and prevented with adequate prophylaxis.

Increasing dietary fibre alone is insufficient (and often unpalatable) in these patients. The most frequently used approach is a combination of a stimulant with a softener, either using a fixed combination such as co-danthramer, or using a stimulant such as senna with a softener or bulking agent such as lactulose.

Nausea and vomiting

Nausea and vomiting are also often multifactorial. The history again will give clues as to whether this is a dysmotility-type dyspepsia with feelings of fullness and bloating, in which prokinetic drugs such as domperidone, metoclopramide or cisapride would be the first-line agents; a motion-induced nausea in which cyclizine, prochlorperazine or hyoscine may be a better choice; or a chemoreceptor trigger-zone-mediated nausea (typically in response to a new drug or a metabolic upset) where haloperidol would be the drug of first choice. In cancer patients who are not receiving chemotherapy or radiotherapy, it is not generally helpful to use the new 5-HT antagonist drugs such as ondansetron.

When nausea and vomiting are present, particularly in association with constipation, it is important to exclude intestinal obstruction and hypercalcaemia. Intestinal obstruction is a relatively common problem in cancer patients. It can occur in up to 6% of all cancer patients, up to 24% with colorectal cancer and up to 42% in ovarian cancer patients. The symptoms most complained about are intestinal colic, aching abdominal pain and vomiting. Absolute constipation is also characteristic.

The surgical approach is clearly indicated in patients who are fit enough, even if the prognosis is relatively poor. A palliative colostomy, ileostomy or gastrostomy can bring dramatic relief and restore well-being and dignity, in time to allow the patient to concentrate on other aspects of living. However, operative mortality is relatively high (12–33%) and morbidity is common, one of the worst complications being enterocutaneous fistulae.

For many patients with advancing cancer, surgical intervention is not feasible (nor desired by the patient). Pharmacological treatment can maintain good relief of symptoms for the majority of these patients. Intestinal colic usually responds well to antispasmodics (hyoscine/atropine/loperamide). The aching abdominal pain responds well to strong opioids. Vomiting can be harder to control completely, although good relief of nausea and reduction of vomiting to once or twice a day should be achievable with haloperidol or methotrime-prazine. Recently there have been reports of reduction in nausea and vomiting with the somatostatin analogue octreotide. However, we would recommend limiting its use to specialist centres until its benefits have been further substantiated.

Hypercalcaemia, which usually presents with nausea, constipation, delirium and thirst, can be treated with good relief of symptoms in many patients with intravenous rehydration and bisphosphonates. Hypercalcaemia has a tendency to relapse and may need repeated treatments at intervals of 2–4 weeks. Regular monitoring of serum calcium is advised after an episode of hypercalcaemia.

Anorexia

Anorexia is common in advancing cancer. If it is associated with nausea, particularly that caused by gastric stasis, simply treating this will sometimes be enough to improve the appetite. Other secondary causes should likewise be treated and explanation given that with decreased activity the appetite often diminishes. Family carers should be instructed to offer the patient small light meals, avoiding strong smells and flavours. If dysphagia is present it is helpful to recruit the assistance of a dietician, who can also advise on the most appropriate high-calorie diet and protein supplementation.

Corticosteroids have been used extensively to stimulate appetite in patients with advancing cancer and there is some evidence to support their use. However, the benefit is usually short-lived in most patients and long-term use brings the risk of serous side effects such as fluid retention, muscle weakness, osteoporosis, skin fragility and candidal infection. More recently there has been substantial evidence that progestogenic drugs such as megestrol may stimulate appetite and produce weight gain at a smaller cost in side effects.

Respiratory symptoms

Respiratory symptoms are found not only in those with primary lung cancer or with secondary lung deposits, but also as a result of the systemic effects of cancer such as anaemia and muscle weakness.

Dyspnoea is the most common respiratory symptom in those with advancing cancer. Again it is important to determine and treat the underlying cause wherever possible. Wherever possible pleural effusions should be aspirated and where they are recurrent pleuradhesis may be indicated. Bronchial obstruction due to tumour may respond well to radiotherapy – either conventional external beam or endobronchial (brachytherapy). Endobronchial laser therapy or stenting is a useful alternative where the tumour is less radiosensitive or the maximum dose has been given, but these options and also brachytherapy are expensive and restricted to a few centres. Chemotherapy or hormonal manipulation may help in selected cases. The treatment of SVC obstruction with either radiotherapy or stenting will also provide substantial palliation, not only of the dyspnoea but also of the discomfort and disability secondary to venous engorgement.

Where present, secondary causes of dyspnoea such as anaemia, ventricular failure, bronchospasm, pericardial effusion, pulmonary embolism and infection should be diagnosed and appropriately treated. Oxygen should be freely available for genuinely hypoxaemic patients or those with underlying airways disease.

Other basic measures should also be introduced at an early stage: attention to sitting and sleeping position, movement of air over the patient's face with a fan or an open window, explanation and reassurance that they will not suffocate.

Drug treatment of dyspnoea principally relies on respiratory sedatives. Opioids are the most frequently used and in contrast to their use in cancer pain it is often most appropriate to prescribe them 'as required'. There is no evidence at present that the nebulized route presents any benefit over the oral route for palliation of dyspnoea with opioids and until more research has been completed it cannot be recommended for routine use outside clinical trials or specialist centres. Benzodiazepines are also commonly used, having an anxiolytic as well as a respiratory depressant effect.

The palliation of cough should also follow the same principles of diagnosis and treatment of cause first, followed by symptomatic treatment if still necessary. Symptomatic treatments can be either directed to increase expectoration (such as physiotherapy or nebulized saline or terbutaline), or to suppress the cough reflex (such as simple linctus or a small dose of opioid). Nebulized local anaesthetics have also been given to suppress the cough reflex with reported benefit, but because of the risk of bronchospasm should only be given under close medical supervision.

The 'death rattle' is a common terminal event due to the pooling of secretions in the trachea. While most patients are unaware of this noise in their semiconscious state, it may cause distress to relatives or patients nearby. Reassurance that the patient is not suffering is essential. Secretions may be diminished with an anticholinergic such as hyoscine given by either subcutaneous bolus or continuous infusion. Initiating this at an early stage will be more successful than waiting until the rattle is distressing. Occasionally repositioning or gentle suction may also be needed.

Other symptoms

It is impossible to cover all common symptoms in this book. Practitioners should have ready access to the numerous texts on symptom control or oncology (see the reading list at the end of the chapter), and should freely consult specialist doctors and nurses, who may give advice over the telephone or arrange to see the patient at home or as an outpatient.

Holistic approach

Although we have dealt with symptoms separately in this chapter it is important to remember that they are often part of a complicated web of distress. When a patient presents with severe pain it may be that it all started as a mild ache. He took some codeine for the ache and it made him constipated and this constipation resulted in overflow diarrhoea and incontinence. In turn this has put a burden on his already distressed family and evoked shame and anger in the patient. These have resulted in a breakdown in communication between him and his wife. In his isolation he has struggled with the question 'why me?' and his spiritual anguish has precipitated guilt and depression, exacerbating the marital disharmony. He cannot talk to his wife about his feelings and the only level on which he can communicate his distress is in talking about his pain.

In adopting an holistic approach to palliative care, it is necessary to consider all aspects as important, but also to acknowledge that at any time one aspect – physical, psychological, social or spiritual – may predominate. It is then necessary to seek help from an appropriately trained practitioner if the problem is beyond one's own professional or personal competence.

Specialist palliative care

The principles of palliative care are simple and should be applied by all clinicians. All doctors should also be competent at basic pain and symptom management. However, rather like asthma care, diabetic care or the management of depression, while much of this care will be provided by primary care services there is also a point at which the simple first-line approaches are inadequate or the non-specialist health-care professionals exhaust their resources. This is the point at which the support of specialist care services should be sought.

The specialist palliative care professionals have advanced training and greater experience and should be aware of the new developments both in management and in services for these patients, which are both expanding at a rapid pace. They are also able to try newer therapies in a controlled environment, increasingly in the context of clinical trials, thus enlarging the knowledge base from which palliative care can be provided.

It is estimated that about 24% of all patients who die of cancer in the UK are seen by a specialist palliative care team. The range of provision varies from area to area but most districts in the UK now have access to community specialist palliative care nurses. There are more than 200 inpatient (hospice) units in the UK with an average of 18 beds per unit. 74% have a daypatient facility and 76% support a home care team. Home care teams (sometimes configured as 'hospice-at-home') vary in composition from purely nursing staff to a full multidisciplinary team including doctors, physical therapists, social workers, psychologists and a range of nursing grades. It is only something approximating to the latter model that can truly provide the full benefits of hospice care at home.

There are an increasing number of palliative care outpatient facilities operating from hospices or hospitals, both as stand-alone clinics and also within combined cancer care clinics. These may develop in the future with 'outreach' clinics placed in the community, which is in keeping with the current trend towards a community bias in health-care provision. Clearly these new approaches, and the more traditional hospice-based model, need to be thoroughly evaluated on both clinical and cost-effectiveness grounds for purchasers and providers with independent budgets to make reasoned choices for their patients' care.

The mark of competent health-care professionals is that they not only provide good palliative care to all their patients but are also aware of their own limitations and seek specialist advice when appropriate. Patients should not be left to suffer without having been offered access to the resources of specialist palliative care services.

Summary

- Palliative care is concerned with holistic care of physical, psychological, social and spiritual problems of people with incurable cancer and other progressive diseases.

- It depends on multidisciplinary teamwork between doctors, nurses, professions allied to medicine, social work and chaplaincy.

- Palliative care can be delivered in the community by the primary care team, but many patients will also benefit from the expertise of specialists working in hospices, hospitals and community teams.

- Good symptom control requires accurate and detailed assessment, frequent monitoring and an awareness of side effects and interactions.

- The WHO guidelines on pain control should be used for the management of cancer pain.

References

1   World Health Organization (1990) *Cancer Pain Relief and Palliative Care. Report of a WHO Expert Committee. WHO Technical Report Series 804.* WHO, Geneva.

Further reading

Cancer Relief Advisory Group (1995) *Helpful Essential Links to Palliative Care.* Centre for Medical Education, Dundee.

Doyle D, Hanks G W and MacDonald N (1993) *Oxford Textbook of Palliative Medicine.* Oxford University Press, Oxford.

Hanks G W (1994) *Palliative Medicine: Problem Areas in Pain and Symptom Management.* Cold Spring Harbor Laboratory Press, New York.

Regnard C and Hockley J (1995) *Flow Diagrams in Advanced Cancer and Other Diseases.* Edward Arnold, London.

Twycross R (1995) *Introducing Palliative Care.* Radcliffe Medical Press, Oxford.

8

Supportive and shared care

J Owen and C Black

Introduction

The diagnosis of cancer used to confer an immediate and irrefutable death sentence upon the patient. The scope of the technology available today has now made that chilling prognosis untrue. The range of treatments available and the advances in the detection of cancer at an early stage have in essence defined cancer as a chronic condition.[1]

Chronic illnesses are 'characterized by remissions and exacerbations and slowly progressive physical changes'.[2] Patients with cancer are now living longer, but that period of life is often punctuated by ill health. Therefore it may be seen that as the illness slowly progresses the patient makes increasing demands on the health-care system, with an increasing need for continuing support and care.

Professionals caring for the cancer patient should view care as a continuous process whether it takes place in the hospital or the community setting. Care differs only in the nature of the illness and the treatment being given: in other words, is active treatment being given (with either curative or palliative intent), or is symptom control and maintenance of quality of life until death the primary aim of that care?

Supporting the patient through their cancer journey requires the skills of all the members of the multidisciplinary team in conjunction with patient and family. If care is to be a truly continuous process, then the importance of sharing the care between the hospital and community setting has to be acknowledged.

This chapter discusses the needs of the cancer patient and his family in the hospital and community setting, and the role of the health-care professionals in meeting those needs. It will also discuss some outcomes of care, and ways in which care can be facilitated between hospital and community. It will go on to examine some of the most common problems that cancer patients experience at home and ways in which they can be resolved.

The impact of cancer on the patient and family

Changes in one's situation, or an accumulation of change events which may induce threat, loss or challenge, are potentially stressful.[3] The diagnosis and treatment of cancer mean that the patient and their family have to undergo many adjustments, some very quickly, others over a period of time. A diagnosis of cancer is to many people the realization that their worst nightmares have come true. Cancer provokes more apprehension and horror than any other disease.[4]

The patient is confronted by his own mortality, the family by the potential loss of a loved one. There is fear of pain, illness, and death without dignity. Treatment invokes its own horrors with potentially distressing side effects and variable response rates. If the patient is a child other siblings may be ignored as the parents' attention is focused solely on the sick child. If the patient is a breadwinner, how will the family cope financially with loss of income which may be long-term or permanent? Who will look after the children in the event of death? How will the partner and other family members cope with illness and death? How will colleagues and friends react? Cancer patients have been shown to adjust to their diagnosis less well than people with other illnesses.[5]

The role of the health care professional in supporting the patient and his family at this time is complex and variable. Psychological adjustment to illness may take many months, and the patient and family may require intense support during this time. However, the hospital doctor or nurse may not be the pivotal person in helping to facilitate the process of adjustment to the illness and its treatment. Cancer patients see many hospital personnel during their periods of treatment, and it is difficult to form attachments when there may not be any continuity of staff between one hospital visit and the next. The role of the community health team should not therefore be under-rated.

Patients have often known their GP for many years, and may place great faith in what s/he says or does; the GP is usually the first person the patient discusses their fears of cancer with. Community nurses have a caseload and a small team working with them; there are not so many different faces visiting. The community Macmillan nurse maintains contact throughout (once referral has been made).

The important role of the hospital team in aiding adaptation and support to the cancer patient should not be minimized or dismissed, but it needs to be acknowledged that cancer patients spend most of their lives in the home care setting, broken usually by only short admissions to hospital.[6] Therefore most of the cancer patient's psychological and physical adjustment to cancer takes place outside that environment – at home.

Maintaining the continuity of supportive and shared care

For care to be viewed as a continuum between hospital and home it requires planning. It has been argued that discharge planning should be considered at the time of admission to hospital.[7] All too often hospital staff underestimate the effect that imminent discharge may have upon the patient and family. If the patient is relatively self-caring then discharge is viewed as a release from the confines of the sick role which all too often is still imposed on patients; but if the patient is less well, then there will be fears of how well they will cope without the additional support of the hospital in maintaining pain control, pressure area care, mobility and so on.

Today, discharge planning is not the sole responsibility of the nursing staff as all the members of the multidisciplinary team from medical staff to pharmacist play a part. The nurse, however, tends to take on the role of coordinator in this process. The nurse will be involved in all aspects of the patient's care, both physical and psychological, as well as facilitating adjustment to changed circumstances.

It is often the nurse who will refer the patient to the appropriate member of the health-care team, for example the medical social worker who can discuss with the patient the grants and allowances to which they may be entitled. The medical social worker will look at the patient's home circumstances and discuss with the patient how these may be altered to fit their circumstances, for example altering steps to make a ramp for a wheelchair, or something as simple as having a telephone installed. The physiotherapist may be involved in improving mobility or teaching the family how to lift or turn the patient. The dietician is involved in discussing diet and nutritional needs, and involving the community care team if the patient is receiving total parenteral nutrition (TPN) at home. The medical staff are involved in coordinating continuing treatments (such as home oxygen), and the pharmacist in discussing appropriate drug interventions.

Once discharge has been planned, the community care team need to be informed in an effective way. One way to achieve this is through the community liaison nurse, who acts as the interface between hospital and home. S/he can be instrumental in planning safe and appropriate discharge if s/he is utilized correctly. Often the community liaison nurse is only notified on the day of discharge; it makes better sense to notify her or him before that date so that community care facilities can be set up. Even if the hospital does not have the services of a community liaison nurse, discharge can be effectively planned and carried out. The main key to its success is communication.

The role of communication in discharge planning

Information to the community care team regarding all aspects of a patient's care is vital if care is to be continued appropriately. In the words of Houlton: 'Relevant, effective communication between hospital and community (nurses) is the only efficient way to ensure continuity of care for patients and their families'.[8] The use of a discharge sheet (Figure 8.1) is one way to promote this process. The discharge sheet serves as a guide to care and treatment received in hospital, and the patient's needs after discharge. It should discuss the patient's and family's understanding of the illness and future care intentions. The discharge sheet should be written in collaboration with the patient and his family, and if possible the community care team made aware of its contents before discharge. All too often the community care staff are unaware of the patient's needs until they perform a home visit, and the information on the discharge sheet may be inadequate to meet the health care professional's needs.

Other aspects of hospital care such as care plans and treatment information sheets could be sent home with the patient to back up the information given on the discharge sheet. If the patient is on a clinical trial (which often involves unlicensed drugs), a copy of the patient information sheet and a list of potential side effects would do much to allay community staff's fears regarding the treatment. It is important that GPs are aware of discharge and medical care required. Discharge summaries from the hospital take a varying length of time to reach the GP, sometimes as long as 98 days.[9] Liaison with the GP by telephone or fax is essential if a home visit is required shortly after discharge.

Communication, however, is a two-way process, and it is just as important that the primary health-care team communicate effectively with hospital staff prior to admission. All too often an aspect of care has changed in between hospital admissions, and hospital staff are rarely made actively aware of this. Changes could include new or increased medication, different wound dressings or changed dietary needs. The patient and their family are not always aware of why changes have taken place. Hospital staff may therefore undo all the care that has been given in the community due to lack of information. This leads to feelings of frustration in the community staff, and confusion over appropriate care when the patient is discharged home once more.

Common care issues for the cancer patient at home

Stair and McNally identified the following groups as people with cancer who could benefit from home care:[10]

DISCHARGE/TRANSFER OF PATIENTS   G.2066

Date of Transfer	Unit No.
	SURNAME Mr./Mrs./Miss
Date of Admission	FIRST NAMES
	AGE (Years) Date of Birth
NEXT OF KIN—Name	HOME ADDRESS
Address	

Relationship   Tel. No.

DISCHARGE ADDRESS (if different)

Next of kin informed of transfer?   YES/NO

Diagnosis (Complete only for inter hospital transfers)

GENERAL PRACTITIONER
ADDRESS

Outpatient Appointment   Ambulance Ordered   YES / NO

From:—	To:—	OTHER SERVICES NOTIFIED
.... WARD		Health Visitor
.... HOSPITAL		Home Help
.... CONSULTANT		Social Worker
		Other

NURSING CARE — Tick Appropriate Box

Complete Bed Rest	Alert	SPECIAL DIET — Details
Ambulant without help	Disorientated	
,, with 1 nurse	Disorientated at night	
,, more than 1 nurse	**PRESSURE AREAS**	
Non Ambulant		MEDICATION — State drug names etc.
Out for bedmaking	Healthy Red	
	Broken	
Continent		
Incontinent of urine	Affected Area.................................	
Incontinent of faeces	Treatment	
Indwelling catheter		

NURSING REQUIREMENTS — at time of Discharge/Transfer

OTHER COMMENTS (e.g. pre-existing conditions, allergies, appliances, attendances at other treatment centres)

Please return Inter-Hospital Transfer only	NOTES	
	X-RAYS	

Signature...Designation.................................

Figure 8.1: Discharge sheet.

- those with advanced disease requiring symptom control

- those with treatment-related self-care deficiencies, e.g. vascular access devices

- those with treatment-related side effects

- those requiring active treatment at home, e.g. immunotherapy injections.

All the above are common problems in cancer patients, but, if dealt with correctly, they may have a minimal effect on the person's quality of life.

Assessment of an individual's homecare needs should begin in the inpatient or clinic setting, and be communicated promptly and effectively to the relevant members of the home care team so that a nursing care plan can be formulated before the patient develops any problems. For example, a patient having cisplatin chemotherapy may develop delayed nausea and vomiting, and the nursing team needs to be aware of this so that assessments and education can be planned and implemented appropriately.

Whilst written information and care plans may be shared between the hospital and the home, it should be remembered that 'elaborate and lengthy care plans have little or no place in the home. Simplicity and practicality are the nurse's guides upon which educational efforts are based'.[11]

Symptom control in advanced disease

Pain management

Home is the most common setting for ongoing pain management. Regimens may be established in a hospital setting, but it is within the home that they must be implemented and adapted to reflect the changing condition of the patient. Successful pain management can only be achieved by collaboration between the patient, family, home care team and the hospital.

Patients may require several different types of analgesic in order to control their pain fully (Table 8.1).

Many patients require opioids in order to control their pain, and in some circumstances these may need to be given via a subcutaneous pump (e.g. in case of vomiting, malabsorption etc.). In this situation the nurse will be required to visit daily to refill the pump, assess the patient's level of pain relief, and adjust the pump rate accordingly. She will also need to check the site of the infusion for redness and pain, and change it if necessary.

Grade of pain	Analgesic	Side effects
1: requires PRN low-strength analgesics	Aspirin Paracetamol	Gastrointestinal irritation Liver damage
2: requires regular low-strength analgesics	Aspirin and codeine Paracetamol and codeine	As above, and constipation
3: requires regular medium-strength analgesia	Pethidine Dihydrocodeine	Respiratory depression, nausea Constipation, nausea, depression
4: requires regular strong analgesia	Morphine Diamorphine Methadone	Nausea, respiratory depression, constipation As above Respiratory depression, cumulative effect, mildly constipating

Table 8.1:　Analgesics and pain control

Infusion pumps may also contain the antiemetics which should be given prophylactically with high doses of opioid drugs.

Constipation

A common side effect of opioid analgesics, constipation, can cause many problems for the individual such as nausea, vomiting and confusion. The home care team are able to help to prevent this problem by education and support. It is important to realize that even patients who are not eating should, from a physical and psychological point of view, still have their bowels opened regularly. Failure to achieve this can lead to the development of problems for patients and carers.

The patient should be encouraged with fluids and a high-fibre diet, but aperients should be used if needed, and these should always be given prophylactically with high doses of opioid analgesics. Suppositories should be used as needed, and if these are not effective then an enema may be required. If the patient is very constipated then an arachis oil enema may be given at night, followed the next morning by a phosphate enema. This often has dramatic results and brings much relief for all concerned.

Nutritional therapy

Cancer patients often focus on any weight loss that they may experience and, for this reason, often focus on their nutritional needs. Home management may vary from education on balanced nutrition to the administration of enteral feeds. The key to successful nutritional management is patient motivation, family support and continued monitoring.

Treatment-related self-care deficiencies

Vascular access devices

When an individual is undergoing chemotherapy and requires regular venous access, it is often preferable to insert a venous access device such as a Hickman line, Broviac or Port-a-cath. This enables long-term venous access, negates the problem of peripheral access, and can be easily managed at home.

Most central venous access catheters are sited with their tip in the superior vena cava or right atrium of the heart. Entry is most commonly by the subclavian vein, but the internal or external jugular vein or the brachiocephalic vein can be used. The procedure is becoming more common, and may now be performed under a local anaesthetic and so the patient may be discharged home the next day.

They will have two sutures: one at the entry and one at the exit site. These are usually removed at 10 and 14 days, respectively, after line insertion. The exit site usually requires re-dressing every 4–7 days, and the line should be flushed weekly. It is very important that the home care team and the ward liaise closely to ensure that care remains consistent throughout.

Treatment-related side effects

Nausea/vomiting

With the development of modern drugs, such as the 5-HT$_3$ antagonists, chemotherapy- and radiotherapy-induced nausea and vomiting are becoming more controllable. The number of patients receiving their treatment on an outpatient basis continues to increase, and so the homecare team has an important role to play in ensuring that the individual is not experiencing undue side effects.

The following chemotherapy drugs are highly emetogenic:

• cisplatin

• dacarbazine

- high-dose melphalan.

The following are moderately emetogenic:

- carboplatin

- cyclophosphamide

- epirubicin

- actinomycin D

- ifosfamide

- doxorubicin.

Antiemetics should be given intravenously prior to chemotherapy. The most commonly used include metoclopramide and cyclizine, but these are often most effective when given in combination with other drugs. A common regimen is:

Haloperidol – 3 mg orally
Lorazepam – 2 mg orally   } prior to chemotherapy
Dexamethasone – 8 mg intravenously.

Patients are also given metoclopramide to take home.

If very emetogenic drugs are to be given, or the patient has a history of vomiting, then $5HT_3$ antagonists such as granisetron or ondansetron may be used. If there are further problems, then dexamethasone may be added to the regimen.

It is also important to remember that nausea and vomiting may be anticipatory, and so an antianxiolytic may be more effective than an antiemetic. The home care team should pass such information to the hospital if they feel that the patient is unnecessarily anxious about their treatment.

Bone marrow suppression

This is the most common treatment-related toxicity, and may be regarded as a sign that the chemotherapy is being effective. It can manifest itself in problems such as neutropenia, thrombocytopenia or anaemia.

The hospital may decide to monitor the patient with regular blood counts, but if the home care team feel that the patient may have a problem it may be advantageous to perform an urgent full blood count at home prior to referring back to the hospital. It is important to request a differential so that the neutrophil count may be checked.

If any results are abnormal then the home care team should contact the hospital for advice. It may be a matter of simply prescribing antibiotics; alternatively the hospital may wish to admit the patient for observation, or to administer a blood transfusion or intravenous antibiotics, etc.

A patient who is neutropenic can develop septicaemia and die within hours. It is vital that the home care team contact the hospital at any time if they have any queries or worries at all.

The role of haematopoietic growth factors (following page) in preventing neutropenic sepsis is now being established.

Active treatment at home

Shared-care protocols

The type of therapies offered to cancer patients today mean that treatment for the illness no longer ends at discharge. Therapy may be continued or even initiated at home. This has required a shift of emphasis from solely hospital-based care to care that is 'shared' between the hospital and community settings.

Shared care between hospital and community is not a new concept, it has occurred as a response to an unfulfilled need of a group of patients receiving active treatments at home (usually some form of immunotherapy, or continuous infusional chemotherapy). Activating a shared-care protocol has resource implications (especially in the community) and implications for clinical accountability. Until recently shared-care protocols have been very much a 'gentlemen's agreement', hospital-initiated and controlled but funded by GPs.

The Department of Health has now recognized the importance of formalized shared care agreements in their Executive Letter EL (95)5 *Purchasing High-Tech Health Care for Patients at Home* which was implemented on 1 April 1995. This will remove funding of home care therapy treatments from GPs (through FP10 prescriptions) to providing health care through a formal contract between purchasers and providers at district level. Treatments will be initiated at the hospital and further supplies arranged either via the hospital or the supplier of the treatment directly.

This will also clarify the issue of clinical responsibility for this group of patients. Responsibility will now rest with the provider, but the purchaser (who may be a fundholding GP) and the community care team will still need to be familiar with the implications of therapy.

Shared care protocols will develop and enhance patient care whilst promoting the philosophy of continuity of care between hospital and community.

Immunotherapy

This is the most common type of active anti-cancer or supportive therapy given in the home. Two agents are routinely given, either the biological response-modifier interferon or a haematopoietic growth factor such as granulocyte-colony stimulating factor (G-CSF).

Interferon is given as treatment for melanoma and renal cell carcinoma, either singly or in combination with other anti-cancer therapy. It is often given as a subcutaneous injection three times per week (usually Monday, Wednesday and Friday). Side effects are usually mild, but can include 'flu-like' symptoms such as muscle pain (myalgia) and shivering alleviated by paracetamol or a NSAI drug. It is usual to try and give the injection as late in the day as possible so that the patient can 'sleep through' the problem time. It is also important to try and give the injection at the same time every day.

The important role of haematopoietic growth factors in decreasing the risk of septicaemia by lessening the severity and duration of neutropenia in patients undergoing chemotherapy has been recognized in the last few years by clinicians. This has led to their increased use. Patients receiving growth factor therapy may do so at home. This requires the home care team to be aware of the reasons for prescription, the correct treatment schedule and the most common side effects associated with their use.

Continuous infusional chemotherapy

Infusional chemotherapy as part of ongoing cancer therapy is becoming more popular. Patients will receive most or all of their treatment at home. This has implications for the home care team and requires close collaboration with the hospital. This type of treatment is the most likely to form part of a shared-care protocol in cancer care. The most commonly prescribed regimen is continuously infused fluorouracil (5FU) for advanced colorectal cancer.

Conclusion

The majority of cancer patients will be at home for most of the time they have their illness. Throughout the progression of their illness their treatment and needs will change. In order for these changes to occur smoothly and without detriment to the patient, it is vital that the hospital and the home care team are in regular contact with each other. Consultants and junior medical staff need to inform GPs of treatment changes and the resulting potential problems, and nurses need to be aware of the physical and emotional needs of the individual. Only by communicating effectively with each other – either through shared-care protocols, or in an informal but no less important way – can we hope to achieve and maintain a high quality and continuity of care for these patients wherever their care may occur. To summarize:

- cancer has a major impact on the patient and the family

- continuity of care between hospital and home is essential

- effective communication has a vital role in discharge planning

- there are common care issues for the cancer patient at home
  - symptom control in advanced disease
  - minimization of treatment-induced toxicities
  - continuation of treatment under a shared-care protocol.

References

1   Traynor B (1992) Quality of life. *J Canc Care.* **1**: 35–40.

2   Shafer K *et al.* (1979) *Medical Surgical Nursing.* C V Mosby, St Louis.

3   Lazarus R and Folkman S (1984) *Stress, Appraisal and Coping.* Springer, New York.

4   Fallowfield L (1990) *The Quality of Life: The Missing Measurement in Health Care.* Souvenir Press (Educational and Academic), London.

5   McCorkle R and Germoni B (1984) What nurses need to know about home care. *Oncol Nurs Forum.* **11**: 63–9.

6   Haylock P J (1993) Home care for the person with cancer. *Home Health-care Nurse.* **11(5)**: 16–28.

7   Turton P and Barnett J (1981). In *Going Home: A Guide for Helping the Patient on Leaving Hospital* (eds J Simpson and R Levitt), Longman, London.

8   Houlton E (1988). In *Oncology for Nurses and Health Care Professionals,* 2nd edn (eds R Tiffany and P Webb), Harper and Row, London.

9 Gilmore N, Bruce N and Hunt M (1976) *The Work of the Nursing Team in General Practice.* Council for the Education and Training of Health Visitors, London.

10 McNally J C (1990) Home care. In *Cancer Nursing: Principles and Practice,* 2nd edn (eds S Groenwald, M Frogge, M Goodman *et al.*), p. 1403–31. Jones and Bartlett, Boston.

11 Maloney C and Preston F (1992) An overview of home care for patients with cancer. *Oncol Nurs Forum.* **19**: 75–80.

Further reading

Blecke C (1989) Home chemotherapy safety procedures. *Oncol Nurs Forum.* **16**: 719–21.

Hileman J, Lachey N and Hassanein R (1992) Identifying the needs of home caregivers of patients with cancer. *Oncol Nurs Forum.* **19**: 771–7.

Sansivero G and Murray S (1989) Safe management of chemotherapy at home. *Oncol. Nurs. Forum.* **16**: 711–13.

Taylor E, Ferrel B, Grant M *et al.* (1993) Managing cancer pain at home: the decisions and ethical conflicts of patients, family caregivers, and homecare nurses. *Oncol Nurs Forum.* **20**: 919–27.

9

Ethical issues

A G O Crowther

Introduction

Since the human organism exhibits an infinite range of reactions which are moulded and are indeed continually evolving and changing through life, the ethical issues that arise from cancer patients are richly variable. The patient's reactions to a given set of circumstances will depend, to some extent, on their genetic make-up, but will also be considerably influenced and developed as a result of the effects from innumerable external factors, which may be thought of as the patient's total environment. It is this multifactorial influence on human behaviour and reaction to circumstances that makes man such a complicated and unique being.

To make the whole issue more interesting, not to say complicated, we must accept that both the family and the friends of the patient react to a given situation as a result of these same influences. Similarly the members of the caring professions that the patient and those close to them go to for advice, treatment and support, are a complicated summation of an infinite number of influences which include their previous professional experience, education and training. Following these considerations it might seem remarkable that ethical issues are able to be addressed at all, let alone with any satisfactory conclusions. It is important to remember that in ethics there is no black or white: it is all about various shades of grey.

We as a society, however, must not turn away from the subject of ethics since it should be thought of as a practical way of organizing our way of living and dying.

Even the World Health Association's 1964 Declaration of Helsinki, which addressed the consent to medical procedures, hinted strongly at the difficulties when it stated: 'if at all possible, consistent with patient psychology, the doctor should obtain the patient's freely given consent after the patient has been given a full explanation'.[1]

Working in the community, health-care workers are not exempt from ethical issues: in fact they are often at the front line of decisions with cancer patients and their families. They often know the circumstances of the patient and the family far more comprehensively and intimately than hospital colleagues or those working in other institutions, e.g. hospices, nursing homes or residential homes. This often means that patient and family will turn to them for ethical guidance, which in turn may create serious dilemmas for them when the hospital's advice and guidance is somewhat different. Good communication between professionals goes some way to alleviate this problem but in the real world this is not always achievable, not least because of time restraints.

General considerations

Here are a few guidelines which may help to clarify the ethical situation.

- Who is the person we are talking about? Is it the person now? Is it the person when younger? Is it the person at other times in their life?

- Who, if anyone, has the right to speak for the patient who cannot speak or otherwise communicate, or is the patient so overwhelmingly anxious that they are unable to handle the situation? Is there a spokesperson? Is the next of kin relevant?

- If there is such a spokesperson, how does s/he begin to understand how the patient feels? What knowledge or skills does that person have to assist with decisions affecting the patient?

- Which moments in the past should be considered when we handle the ethical issues? Admission to a hospice or other health care establishment is an ethical consideration where assumptions are taken; the patient then enters a different area of life.

- What are the ethical guidelines within medical care with regard to aggressive medical technology? How do we keep a balance of care for the patient?

- What guidelines do we have with regard to the use of drugs which are known to cause extra sedation? We must consider these guidelines to help us with such decisions.

To try and understand further how complicated the subject of medical ethics is, and yet to try and bring some order into the subject, in recent years a 'four principles plus scope' approach has been developed.[2] Put at its simplest, this suggests that whatever our personal philosophy, politics, religion, moral theory or life stance, we will find no difficulty in committing ourselves to four moral principles plus a reflective concern regarding their scope of application. The four moral principles are:

- autonomy (self-rule)
- beneficence
- non-maleficence
- justice.

Beneficence with non-maleficence refers to the obligation of medicine to provide net medical benefit to patients with minimal harm. As for justice, this can be sub-divided into three further categories:

- distributive – the fair distribution of limited resources
- rights – respect for peoples' rights
- legal – the respect of morally acceptable laws.

Scope allows for a balance to be taken between the above four categories when applied to a particular circumstance, in order to avoid possible conflict.

Inevitably ethical practice is constantly changing and evolving with time. What was not acceptable ethical practice a few years ago may now be quite acceptable; equally, what is acceptable practice now may become not so in the future. Therefore when we are handling these issues we, the health-care professionals, are part of that evolutionary process so that we may, by our efforts, be unwittingly pushing boundaries forward. This is desirable and right because nothing in this area of life stands still.

From the patient's viewpoint

In a further attempt to understand the ethical issues surrounding the patient with cancer let us look at three main areas of importance, starting with the patient, who has rights, needs, demands and sometimes obsessions. Patients increasingly have improved knowledge of medical matters but we should remember this is often sketchy and media-biased. Also it is frequently very different in application when the person with that knowledge becomes the patient. We should not forget that even doctors, who can be expected to have reasonable medical knowledge, often react in unpredictable and unreliable ways when they become the patient.

The professional can tease out the patient's medical knowledge and, if appropriate, build on it to give that patient a better understanding of the situation. Perhaps the patient's rights are more easy to understand than his or her needs, which require careful consideration and negotiation to stand a chance of getting it right for that individual at that particular time. The demands may be easy or totally impossible; if they are the latter, the health-care professional needs to take a careful look at this area and then fairly and firmly try to guide the patient towards more realistic demands. We need to acknowledge areas of obsession and, if appropriate, re-channel these into useful attitudes; a caring family or friends can often help considerably.

From the family members' viewpoint

The patient's family and close friends also have needs and demands. These have to be secondary to those of the patient but nevertheless must be acknowledged. If the needs are similar to those of the patient then it is all relatively easy, but on occasions these are different and we must try to bring them closer to those of the patient. This will result in them reinforcing one another rather than achieving a dilution of need, which in turn inevitably leads to resignation or conflict.

The demands of relatives, similarly, if different from those of the patient, can be difficult to handle. In my experience they frequently stem from a combination of not understanding what the patient is trying to handle, that the patient feels ill while the relative feels generally well and also that they cannot bear the pain of potentially losing their relative or even of seeing them ill and losing ground. This can result in a demand for a continuation of treatment. These relatives can eventually become quite unrealistic and, for their own sakes – particularly with regard to the immediate future and also the forthcoming bereavement – must be guided firmly to a greater realism. The resulting understanding and acceptance will keep them in their support of the patient. The achievement of this realism can be difficult and time-consuming but it is important and of considerable help to all concerned. It can also be professionally satisfying when the results of these efforts to bring about more realism are seen.

From the professional carers' viewpoint

Doctors and other health-care workers have a different set of moral issues to contend with, starting with the communication of bad news to a patient and family. No one enjoys this and it is often done badly. Increased training in communication skills is improving the situation but again it requires that scarce commodity – time – to achieve the best for patients and families. Many doctors have particular difficulty since they still feel that not being able to cure the patient is a sign of failure. Continued and further training at medical student level and during the pre-registration appointments may help in this area.

Some investigations are unpleasant and frightening for patients, and a judgment of the benefits for doing the test as against the disadvantages of not doing it must be made, remembering that each patient is unique.

The patient can be subjected to modern treatments (e.g. drugs, surgery and/or radiotherapy) and the appropriateness of such must be considered and evaluated. The patient and family must be involved in the decision-making process, without actually being forced to take the decisions themselves.

One of the most difficult decisions in the acute sector of health care is when to change from active to palliative treatment or just supportive care. With modern techniques it can be difficult not to try these on patients but, after reasonable discussion of the position, patients and families will generally make it plain what they want. Although it all takes time, this discussion should take into account as many factors as possible, ideally including the views of the primary health-care team who know the patient and family.

In summary, from the clinical standpoint there are two complementary systems of treatment which may often overlap: one system is concerned with eliminating a curable disease and the other with relieving the symptoms resulting from the relentless progress of an incurable disease.[3] There must be openness, interchange and overlap between the two systems so that the patient receives continuous and appropriate care. The patient should not be subjected to aggressive treatment that offers no real hope of curing or controlling the disease and which may only cause further distress. However, the clinician must also be on the alert for any shifts that may occur in the course of a patient's terminal illness, which may result in him becoming a candidate for active treatment.

Patients can suffer not only from inappropriate active care but also from inept terminal care.

There is also the question of moving forward and advancing medicine with clinical research. Ethics committees have the responsibility for approving all clinical trials carried out in the NHS. Such committees have Department of Health-approved membership and are composed of both medical and lay members. Pharmaceutical companies cannot have direct contact with any of the ethics committees; submission of any research trial protocol must be to the local committee by the principal investigator – usually but not exclusively a doctor. If a trial protocol is altered during the trial it is necessary to inform the ethics committee, at the least via the chairperson; s/he will decide whether the entire study has to be revised or whether, if it is a relatively minor alteration, the trial can continue without delay.[4]

In recent years there have been problems of inconsistency between various ethics committees, so during 1994 the Department of Health sent out three documents to all local research ethics committees (LRECs). The aim was to assist and standardize working practices with various guidelines: e.g. *Standards for Local Research Ethics Committees – a Framework for Ethical Review* (available from Mr S. Goulding, Department of Health, Wellington House, 133–155 Waterloo Road, London SE1 8UG), *Standard Operating Procedures for LRECs* and *Using Standards for LRECs* (available on disk from Mrs C Bendall, McKenna & Co., 160 Aldergate Street, London EC1A 4DD, priced £10.00).

Clinical staff still have ethical decisions to make with regard to entering or offering to enter any given patient to a trial. These are not and cannot be made by ethics committees. Some patients are very keen to enter such trials, which may give them strength and increased determination to cope with their disease. Others being entered on a trial will develop increased levels of anxiety and fear. Just to add to the imponderables, the patient's and relatives' attitudes to being on a trial may alter if and when the disease progresses. All clinical staff must be alert to these feelings throughout their contact with the patient and family so as to be aware of any attitude changes and to be ready to act as guide or mentor to that patient.

Budgetary constraints

Doctors should not be swayed by their understandable desire to try out new treatments, nor by the growing pressure to publish. A more serious problem is the question of resources. There is not an infinite amount of money for treatments which are forever advancing; this progress is good, but is frequently expensive. So not only do clinicians have to balance the ethics of persuading or offering a particular patient a treatment option: there is also the consideration of whether the cost is justified, having acknowledged the likely outcome. Whether these decisions should be made by the clinicians or the purse-holding administration is an ever-present dilemma. Common sense generally prevails, but distortion by the media does not help anyone. Perhaps society as a whole has to address this issue, because it involves treating or not treating on account of age and other social criteria. In the meantime, good communication at the clinical level with an understanding of good general clinical care for the patient usually resolves most of these dilemmas. This is an area where many of the problems do not arise when the clinicians and the administrators have a good working relationship rather than an 'us-and-them' attitude.

It is easy to say we should not use aggressive therapies with our treatments, but as a result of these a good proportion of patients with acute leukaemia, for example, can now be cured or at least given lengthy remission. Similarly some patients with carcinoma of the bladder die during or soon after a radical course of radiotherapy, but many are cured; we tend to forget the cures and only remember the distress caused to the other unfortunate patients. There are many other examples of particular cancers where aggressive treatment results in cure or reasonable remission. However, the criticism from relatives and patients who have not responded to the treatment and have also had their quality of life prejudiced as a result of that treatment is painful for the clinical staff. The 'retrospectoscope' is a very difficult instrument to handle and yet we must be mature enough to absorb its findings so as to help with future ethical issues. All doctors and nurses at times have to walk a tightrope between overtreatment and neglect; the overall and eventual comfort of the patient must come first. We have all heard of 'the art and science of medicine' and perhaps many ethical issues arrive from this double thrust. The patients and relatives are right to want more information, and it is often difficult to admit that the clinical staff do not necessarily have all the answers. It may be that many ethical issues arise as a result of a real shift by health care workers towards the science of medicine, this compounded by an unrealistic shift towards the science by society within which are our patients and their relatives. The art of medicine, particularly communication skills and other ways of behaving towards patients and families, is a vital area in the unravelling of the many and various ethical issues that we meet in cancer patients.

On the other hand, perhaps this is why this whole area of health care is full of such interest, challenge, stimulus and professional satisfaction; there is a constantly changing situation to be handled. After all, it is said that life itself is a compromise, so we should not expect this area of clinical care to be different. Anyone entering a caring profession takes on the obligation to handle the relevant dilemmas to the best of their ability; we should not therefore turn away from that responsibility.

Summary

The ten indicators regarding ethical issues are as follows.

- Take time with decisions. If a course of action is not obvious it will pay dividends to delay a while. Time is not only a great healer, it is also a valuable aid to assessment in a changing clinical picture.

- Communicate with the patient and relatives/close friends. This takes time and effort but pays handsome dividends.

- Whenever possible involve patients and relatives/close friends in clinical decisions and the reasons for them. If they feel part of the decision-making process they will have greater confidence in the health-care team. They do not take the decisions but are part of the mechanism for making them.

- Be open when discussing situations leading to decisions regarding clinical management, not only with patients and relatives but with other health professionals involved. Secrecy is dangerous and is frequently misunderstood.

- If a decision cannot be reached, do not be too proud to ask for further guidance or a second opinion.

- Remember the patient might be you or someone close to you. It has been said that a clinician should not order something for a patient that they themselves would not have.

- Compromise is generally better than confrontation for everyone concerned.

- In this area of clinical work many answers cannot be definitive (expected progress of disease, cure, speed of spread, time to death etc.). It is important to stress the reasons for the necessary vagueness when asked pertinent questions of this nature. Social factors play an important part in this process of communication.

- Clinical decisions are not cast in stone. Constant review is necessary and, when appropriate and relevant, a change should be made with the knowledge and approval of all those involved (e.g. patient and/or relatives, and other clinical staff).

- Patient autonomy is not an excuse for the professional to opt out of decision-taking. The patient must have adequate information to enable them to be involved in clinical decisions if they so wish. Patients come to us for professional advice; however, many ill or anxious patients want the health professional to make a decision for them. There is a balance to be struck between total patient autonomy and health professional dogmatism, and this is an ethical issue in itself.

- Document the broad outline with the various points considered clearly stated. This is important not only for medicolegal reasons, but also because committing to paper the conclusions and how they were arrived at clears the mind, helps communication (allowing for the written word) and is often vital when discussing issues later.

- All health-care workers must remember they are dealing with fellow human beings and should do so with humility and dignity. We are here for the patient; the patient is not here for us.

References

1   Skegg P D G (1984) *Law, Ethics and Medicine; Studies in Medical Law*. Clarendon Paperbacks, Oxford.

2   Gillon R (1994) Medical ethics: four principles plus attention to scope. *BMJ*. **309**: 184–8.

3   Fulton R and Bendiliger W R (1994) *Death and Identity*. Charles Press, Philadelphia.

4   Ranson P (1994) Ethics approval: the legal aspects. *Good Pract J*. July: 10–11.

10

Psychosocial aspects of cancer and its treatment

T W Noble

Psychological care

Since Hippocrates urged us to 'comfort always', emotional support has been at the core of good medical practice. Whether we can cure or not, comforting is one of our tasks. Traditionally, psychological support has been regarded as part of the art, rather than the science, of medicine and related disciplines. This view allows individual creativity in our day-to-day work; however, there is a danger that we thereby imply that the effectiveness of our support may not be evaluated and therefore never improved. While ever we hold to the mystery around these skills, we may also abdicate our responsibility to fringe or complementary therapists whose methods are similarly unevaluated.

Over the past 25 years the multidisciplinary subspecialty of psycho-oncology has advanced our knowledge considerably and we now have detailed information concerning the psychological toll of cancer and its treatment. Psychiatric morbidity in cancer patients has been well documented and the development and controlled evaluation of therapy to improve the psychological health of cancer patients has been undertaken.

Psychosocial oncology – a review of the case for therapy

When cancer patients are screened by psychiatrists, the incidence of a psychiatric disorder which fulfils the formal criteria for diagnosis is found to be between 25% and 47%. One of the best early studies in 1983 randomly accessed 250 new cancer patients at three centres in the USA: 47% were found to have some psychiatric disorder and of these 85% experienced a disorder with anxiety or depression as the central symptom.[1] The diagnoses made in the patients with a disorder were as follows: adjustment disorder, 68%; major affective disorders, 13%; organic mental syndromes, 8%; personality disorders, 7%; anxiety disorders, 4%. Curiously in this study the three centres' prevalence rates were different: 24%, 46% and 69%.

This raises the question why so few cancer patients are treated for psychiatric problems. Studies in general practice, looking at patients with unrecognized depression, found that they were more likely to have a physical illness than those patients whose depression was recognized, and more likely to have suffered symptoms of depression for longer than one year.[2] It would appear that a long relationship with our patients is not helpful when making the diagnosis of depression.

There seem to be two major reasons why depression goes untreated in cancer patients. First, low mood is understandable and therefore seen as a natural reaction to the patient's predicament ('I would be depressed if I had cancer'). This is a curious attitude when we consider that pain is also a natural consequence of many cancers. We do not say, 'of course he's got pain, he's got cancer'. We prescribe adequate analgesia. The second reason is that the symptoms of depression mimic very closely the debility experienced by cancer patients, particularly when the disease is advanced. Physical symptoms of depression such as poor appetite, loss of weight, changes in sleep patterns, agitation or retardation, fatigue and poor concentration, are all on occasion present in patients with cancer but no affective disorder. Also feelings of anxiety, worthlessness, guilt and intrusive thoughts of death seem highly appropriate given knowledge of the diagnosis.

The case for making the diagnosis and treating depression and anxiety in these patients is made by the evidence that drug therapy is highly effective, even though the depression could be said to be reactive. This has been demonstrated by a randomized placebo-controlled trial of mianserin in 73 depressed women with cancer.[3] The diagnosis of depression is made according to DSM-III (R) criteria. However, many oncologists and general practitioners are reluctant to treat, and feel that a psychiatric label seems to be medicalizing the problem. Perhaps the stigma of mental illness (which cancer patients obviously wish to avoid) contributes to the neglect of emotional symptoms at such a stressful time in their lives. There is also a feeling that patients with cancer are particularly sensitive to the side effects of antidepressant drugs. By and large this problem is best avoided by starting with a low dose, e.g. 25–50 mg of dothiepin or amitriptyline taken at night, and then increasing it after a week or two. The usual maintenance dose for cancer patients is generally lower than that for fit patients with depression, but nevertheless the best results are obtained when the maximum dose that can be tolerated is prescribed. It is my practice to titrate the dose of a sedative antidepressant against the patient's sleep disturbance, with the aim being an unbroken night's sleep without sedation in the morning.

There have been a few trials of counselling in patients with cancer. In one, specially trained nurses saw patients after mastectomy.[4] No effect on anxiety or depression was found at three months, however 12–18 months post-mastectomy, there was a difference between the counselled patients and the controls. 39% of the controls, but only 12% of the counselled group had either an anxiety state, a depressive illness or a sexual problem. This result was thought to have reflected the ability of the counselling nurses to detect and refer patients to psychiatrists when appropriate. 77% of the counselled group were referred but only 15% of the controls obtained psychiatric help in the course of their treatment. The form of counselling used in this trial is a style of good professional communication described by Faulkner and Maguire.[5] However, more involved and intensive models of counselling exist, and in a randomized controlled trial of counsellors trained by Dr Kubler-Ross, which involved developing a relationship, talking freely, reminiscing with the patient, sometimes sitting quietly, encouraging meaningful activities, reducing denial, maintaining hope, and often being present at the time of death, a significant improvement in quality of life measures and depression scores at three months after referral was found.[6] This intervention probably represents the kind of psychological support that will never be available either in primary care or specialist centres within the NHS.

Clearly more work is needed, particularly with patients with advanced cancer, to find which part of the intensive interventions yields the most help. However, simple interventions such as the use of an anxiety management booklet have been effective in the general practice setting, and it would seem reasonable to provide this kind of support for patients with cancer who exhibit an anxiety disorder. The effectiveness of the newer selective serotonin reuptake inhibitors has not yet been extensively evaluated. Early experience is that the side effects are generally better tolerated by patients with cancer, except for a few unfortunate individuals who experience particularly severe GI symptoms or agitation.

Benzodiazapines, usually diazepam, clearly have a place in the management of acute anxiety, but since their benefit seems to wane after a week or two of regular use and there is some evidence to suggest that they reduce individuals' ability to cope or seek appropriate other support, their use is not indicated for long-term anxiety symptoms.

Cognitive behavioural treatment has much to offer, particularly soon after diagnosis and during treatment. A form of brief problem-focused therapy, known as adjuvant psychological therapy, developed by Steven Greer's team, has been shown to reduce anxiety and psychological symptoms at eight weeks and four months after treatment. More fighting spirit, less helplessness and less anxious preoccupation were demonstrated, but depression scores were not significantly altered. Fighting spirit has been associated with a more favourable response to treatment.

Psychological distress and its diagnosis

Anxiety disorders and adjustment disorders may be thought of as part of the medical diagnosis or as understandable reactions; the distinction does not exercise us unduly. The treatment – supportive counselling, relaxation training and symptomatic short-term medication – seems commensurate with the distress, and we do not seem to be taking the step of medicalizing the problem.

The diagnosis of depression for the reasons discussed above is a different matter, and there is always a temptation to make a judgement about the degree of understandability. It may be said that the difference between reactive and endogenous depression is that the former diagnosis is made when the doctor thinks he would be depressed in similar circumstances.

It may not be perfect but at present we have no alternative to making the diagnosis by identifying a syndrome of symptoms according to formal criteria for a major depressive episode. These may be summarized as follows.

Major depressive episode

At least five symptoms should be present most of the day, most days, for two weeks. Symptoms clearly directly due to the physical disease should not be included. The symptoms must include low mood and/or loss of interest or pleasure (anhedonia). Other symptoms to check for are:

- weight or appetite change
- sleep change
- agitation or retardation
- fatigue or loss of energy
- feelings of worthlessness or guilt
- poor concentration

- intrusive thoughts of death or suicidal thoughts.

Organic factors, schizophrenia and normal bereavement reaction discount the diagnosis. Diurnal variation of mood and lack of sexual interest are useful pointers to the diagnosis. Symptoms of anxiety or panic disorder commonly coexist and are a consequence of depression.

The network of support

From the point of view of health workers in primary care, there appears to be abundant provision for cancer patients. Day hospices, Macmillan services and oncological day hospitals seem to cover the demand for places. Perhaps it is the horror and dread which accompanies the prospect of the diagnosis of cancer in us or our family that has led to the development of services in the public, private and voluntary sectors. So many different professionals are involved with the delivery of care to patients with cancer that the network of support may appear, from the patient's perspective, as an unorchestrated rabble of attendants. Although a few (usually elderly) individuals will obtain all the care they require from a GP and a district nurse, the majority will at various times in their illness encounter many diverse disciplines, each with a different method, agenda and priority in the provision of care.

When professional skills complement each other, patients benefit from this multidisciplinary approach, but clearly there is a danger of duplication of work. More often, however, there is a worry that patients will fall between us, and no meaningful communication takes place in a succession of superficial encounters. Consultations concerning cancer, uncertain futures, unpleasant treatments and the prospect of death are difficult. There is no single method or framework which is appropriate to all professionals providing support, so how may we ensure that we provide high quality care and facilitate others in their roles? It is tempting for each of us to believe that we are best placed within the team to understand the suffering of our patient, and coordinate care accordingly. This is a healthy attitude in that it demonstrates commitment to our task, but none of us owns our patients even though we may have known them for many years and have an intimate knowledge of their character. The appearance of conflict between professionals, other than healthy rivalry, leads to a feeling of insecurity and uncertainty about the quality of care in general. This in turn raises the emotional temperature of subsequent consultations and all our jobs seem more difficult. Patients by and large feel best supported when they believe their attendants to be working harmoniously or have some sort of positive professional relationship with each other. There seems to be no substitute for developing familiarity and a good working relationship with colleagues in cancer and primary care.

Giving information to patients

One factor which seems to determine a patient's reaction to their diagnosis and prognosis is the way they learn about their predicament. Patients who are unable to handle information will react by denial or by becoming severely withdrawn. The information is more likely to be assimilated if it is given step by step in manageable amounts. The principles of giving bad news by ascertaining the present state of knowledge, and initially giving vague indications that all is not well, allows patients to indicate their need and capacity to know more serious and detailed knowledge. Further detail is given until the present state of available information is conveyed or the patient indicates they have heard enough from that consultation. The interval between a patient thinking they are well and knowing they will die in the foreseeable future is thereby extended and allows natural adjustment.

The nature of the prognosis is more problematic. It is never right to give an estimate of a patient's longevity without being asked. When we are asked, it is important to know the limitations of our knowledge. Several studies have demonstrated our inability to guess the length of a cancer patient's survival. Even if you are very familiar with the survival curves of your patients, it can be terribly misleading to give a median survival since only a small minority of patients adhere to the median and there are no reliable indicators of an individual's position in the population. We do best by owning up to our inability to predict the future and allow our patients to 'hope for the best and plan for the worst'.

Concerns of cancer patients: loss, fear and anger

At the heart of the skills required to deliver support are those which enable us to communicate effectively. They allow us to pick up concerns which trouble our patients. The starting point of support is the assessment of patients' concerns. This will set the context in order that the nature and severity of a patient's suffering may be understood. It is easy to see that the amount of distress aroused in us by the diagnosis of cancer is a function not only of the prognosis, the prospect of unpleasant treatment, and the disruption of life and work, but also the stage of our lives, including the dependency of our family. Resonances from our past, including how our parents and close relatives coped with illness or bereavement, and the psychological healthiness or otherwise of our early lives, have a bearing on the nature of our suffering. The powerful emotions associated with loss, fear and anger are difficult to discuss meaningfully in the abstract until they are ventilated in the context of a patient's story. It is then easy to empathize and thereby validate patients' concerns. Clarifying and agreeing their problems may be therapeutic in itself. Problem-solving strategies may be helpful with some difficulties.

The number of concerns seems in itself to be a risk factor for psychiatric morbidity. Recently cancer patients with four or more concerns have been shown to be significantly more prone to affective disorder than those with fewer concerns.[7] It is never wise to assume you have heard all the things that may be troubling your patient since some of the most distressed cancer patients express many major concerns, given the chance.

It may be helpful to illustrate the variety and extent of concerns expressed in a patient's problem list. A 52-year-old lorry driver, seen six months after a radical gastrectomy for stomach cancer, who developed a major depressive episode presenting with weight loss, mentioned the following concerns:

- shock of diagnosis

- stress of waiting for surgery

- diarrhoea

- weight loss

- low mood

- lack of energy and inability to live normally

- indwelling nasogastric tube

- sadness at prospect of not seeing grandchild grow up

- impotence

- fear of incontinence

- distress at deaths on the ward.

His depression responded to counselling and tricyclics and there is no sign of recurrence of his cancer three years postoperatively.

Family histories and cancer – two anecdotes

Family histories and myths are sometimes powerful determinants of a patient's behaviour. It is tempting to attribute difficult behaviour to an individual's innate characteristics, but it is often more fruitful to understand the behaviour in the context of a patient's beliefs or assumptions about what is happening. A 60-year-old woman became extremely withdrawn following the removal of a large ovarian tumour. She understood it was malignant and that her future was uncertain. The reaction could be said to be understandable, but the ward staff who dealt with similar situations every week identified her as extremely withdrawn and feared that she was contemplating suicide. The explanation was readily identified by the patient herself, who had lost her mother from cancer of the breast when the patient was ten years old. She had overheard her aunt say 'the girl will get cancer too – she was fed at the breast'. The patient had expected to die of cancer all her life; now it seemed to be coming true. The loss of a parent in early life made her susceptible to a difficult reaction to loss of any sort. Once this kind of story is heard and understood by medical attendants, superstitions can be laid to rest. At least the patient's own children may be freed from the curse and, importantly for the patient, she is understood. Antidepressants are still necessary in order to alleviate her symptoms but the story allows us to unburden her of her fears.

In the same way a victim of sexual abuse as a child, who at 20 years old developed Hodgkin's disease, was particularly anxious and fearful of chemotherapy. The reason was not the hair loss and vomiting but the fact that doctors and nurses came into her hospital side ward at night while she slept. She feared the loss of control and her new vulnerability.

Often patients whom I see describe such a catalogue of bad fortune before and after the diagnosis of cancer, that we are forced to conclude that they would be rather peculiar if they did not show some sign of strain.

Families and their problems

Sometimes a patient's distress can only be understood in the context of their family and their place or role within it. It is possible to identify characteristics of family functioning: supportiveness and ability to resolve conflict seem to protect against psychological morbidity in the cancer patient, whereas hostile and sullen families are more prone to social and psychiatric dysfunction.[8]

Perhaps the family problem in cancer care which give professionals the greatest difficulty is collusion and denial. In the context of the family these two go together. The family's collusion is necessary if a patient's denial is to be tolerated; similarly it is impossible for a family to collude to keep the truth from a patient without denial by the patient at some level.

Professionals have a role in preventing this situation by abandoning the old practice of giving a diagnosis and prognosis to relatives before the patient is told. Relatives naturally want to protect the patient from the additional suffering associated with the knowledge of the diagnosis. Occasionally this has been openly agreed before the news is to be heard, but in the majority of cases it leads to stress and barriers at a very important time. Many doctors now see patients together with their family at the bad news interview, thereby modelling openness and providing a vocabulary for discussion afterwards.

Some patients are generally seen alone, others are seen with their family. The preference of the family may appear to be a problem but it provides information about how the family works and how the patient will be treated as the illness progresses. Spouses, sons and daughters bring their own resonances to the bedside and no one should be surprised when our patients behave differently at visiting time. What is unpredictable is the nature of the difference. Reasoned arguments or appeals to act in what you suppose to be the patient's best interest are usually unfruitful.

In general the key to dealing with a relative's difficulty is to focus on the relative's own suffering from their point of view.

Conclusion

In this short chapter I have attempted to outline some simple guiding principles, supported by research evidence. They may be summarized as follows:

- it is kind to treat psychological suffering like physical suffering – effectively

- the diagnosis of depression should be made on the basis of symptoms

- communication is a clinical skill to be learnt and improved like the rest. Someone in the clinical team needs to be communicating effectively

- information needs to be given in a way which is sensitive to a patient's capacity to cope with it

- the nature and severity of the suffering may be understood in the context of the personal and family history

- the family's difficulties have implications for the reaction of the patient as well as vice versa.

References

1   Derogatis L R, Morrow G R, Fetting J *et al.* (1983) The prevalence of psychiatric disorders among cancer patients. *JAMA.* **249**: 751–7.

2   Freeling P, Rao B M, Paykel E S *et al.* (1985) Unrecognised depression in general practice. *BMJ.* **290**: 1880–3.

3   Costa D, Mogos I and Toma T (1985) Efficacy and safety of mianserin in the treatment of depression of women with cancer. *Acta Psych Scand* (**Suppl 320**): 85–92.

4   Maguire P, Tait A, Brooke M *et al.* (1980) Effect of counselling on the psychiatric morbidity associated with mastectomy. *BMJ.* **281**: 1454–6.

5   Faulkner A and Maguire P (1994) *Talking to Cancer Patients and their Relatives.* Oxford University Press, Oxford.

6   Linn M W, Linn B S and Harris R (1982) Effect of counselling for late stage cancer patients. *Am Canc Soc.* **49**: 1048–55.

7   Harrison J, Maguire P, Ibbotson T *et al.* (1994) Concerns, confiding and psychiatric disorder in newly diagnosed cancer patients: a descriptive study. *Psycho-Onc.* **3**: 173–9.

8   Holland J C and Watson M (eds) (1994) Perceptions of family functioning and cancer. *Psycho-Onc.* **3**, 259–69.

Further reading

Barraclough J (1994) *Cancer and Emotion*, 2nd edn. John Wiley, Chichester.

Buckman R (1992) *How to Break Bad News.* Papermac, London.

Corney R (ed.) (1991) *Developing Communication and Counselling Skills in Medicine.* Routledge, London.

Doyle D, Hanks G W C and MacDonald N (eds) (1993) *Oxford Textbook of Palliative Medicine*. Oxford Medical, Oxford.

Moorey S and Greer S (1989) *Psychological Therapy for Patients with Cancer – A New Approach*. Heinemann Medical, Oxford.

Saunders E and Sykes N (1993) *Management of Terminal Malignant Disease*, 3rd edn. Arnold, London.

Stedford A (1984) *Facing Death*. Heinemann Medical, London.

Watson M (ed.) (1991) *Cancer Patient Care: Psychological Treatment Methods*. BPS, Leicester.

11

Communicating with patients and relatives

A Faulkner

Introduction

Communication in cancer care has been a focus of concern for many years.[1–4] More recently, research has been undertaken that concentrates not on the problems of communication between cancer patients, their families and health professionals, but on whether the necessary skills for effective interaction can be taught and maintained over time.[5] Much of the work undertaken has focused on effective interaction between the patient and doctor or nurse while the patient is in hospital. There are, however, particular issues in the community where the patient is away from the safety of the hospital and often attempting to maintain a normal life while struggling with the many issues raised by living with a diagnosis of cancer. Those who work with patients in the community need to consider the particular problems of interacting with an individual in their own home, and also be aware of particular issues which may be raised for the patient.

The patient at home

When a patient is discharged from hospital, the future care of that patient may well be in their own home and provided by a number of professionals responsible for community care. These will include the general practitioner (GP), the district nurse and the Macmillan nurse, and in advanced cancer there may also be hospice personnel. It may also involve the patient in day care at the hospice or in periods of admission to the hospice for respite care. It can be seen that communication between the health professionals involved is vitally important if the patient is to get coherent care and know where to go to discuss any concerns that may arise.

Home visits

Nurses, particularly, find that visiting a patient in their own home is rather different in terms of communicating and offering help. It is often argued that any health professional who offers help in the patient's own home has to take on the role of visitor and in that role to accept the dynamics of what is going on in the household. This can mean that the television is on, that children are running around, that the cat is wanting to come in or go out, and that various other diversions are taking attention from the patient.

It has to be remembered that any health professional visiting a patient in the home is offering a service to that patient. As such, s/he should negotiate the time of the visit and check that the maximum privacy will be available. This gives the patient the choice of having the nurse or doctor visit when the children are at school or at a time when there will be no other diversions. Since the health professional is offering a service in the patient's home, s/he has a right to ask politely for the television to be switched off and whether there is somewhere the patient and health professional can talk with minimal interruptions. Most patients will accept this as a sign of the importance of the interaction and will make all effort to see that there is some element of privacy in the visit.

If the patient's home is such that privacy is not possible, then it might be better if the patient comes to a health clinic or somewhere away from home, where there will be a chance to talk quietly and privately about the matters of concern to the patient, and indeed to the health professional.

Negotiation

Ideally, before patients are discharged from hospital, they should have some notion of what will happen in terms of follow-up when they get home. Depending on the individual's disease and treatment, the follow-up may be through the clinic, through the general practice or through home visiting. If the follow-up is through home visiting, then the patient should know when the health professional will call and also the approximate length of the visit. If the patient has a telephone, then the health professional can telephone ahead and negotiate a suitable time, when they can meet either in privacy in a quiet room if possible, or at a time of day when the patient will be available and not distracted. In many situations, it may be possible to offer the patient a choice of whether the visit is at home or at the local health clinic or GP practice.

In negotiating follow-up care of cancer patients in the community, family issues are very likely to appear more important than they may have done when the patient was in hospital. For example, the negotiation of access to the patient may be through the informal carer, who may be the patient's partner or parent. It is possible that in this role of carer, the relative or close friend becomes very much more protective of the patient than was possible for them in the hospital setting. They may, for example, wish to set rules about what the health professional discloses on a visit, often wishing a promise that prognosis, particularly, will not be discussed. In such a situation, the health professional will need to negotiate with the relative while pointing out that their role is to meet the patient's needs, including the need for information.

Collusion of this type can often be broken by exploring with the relative why they wish the truth to be withheld from their loved one. Many authors have argued that relatives do not want the truth in the open because they themselves cannot cope with the reality of a serious illness. In fact most relatives, particularly parents, wish to protect their loved one from pain, using collusion as an act of love. Collusion has to be broken with care and with due concern for the person who is carrying the burden of the truth without discussing it with their loved one.

Negotiation with the patient or the carer can aid the value of home visits in that ground rules are set for what the visit is about, when it will take place and how long it will take place for. Then both the patient and the carer and the health professional know the parameters within which they are working.

Patient needs

In order to identify the needs of the patient at home following hospitalization for cancer, it is important to assess the adaptation to the home setting following diagnosis, treatment and aftercare. For example, a patient who had been very stable in hospital following mastectomy told the community nurse:

> 'It was OK when I was in hospital, we were all in the same boat, but now I'm home, they expect me to be just as I was before and I'm tired and frightened and I don't know what to do.'

This reaction to coming home is not uncommon. Many cancer patients, for example, have body-image problems. In hospital with other patients these are far less important than on the return to home, where partners become involved in perhaps seeing an unsightly scar or a stoma. Many patients find difficulties with their relationships on returning home because they try to hide their new reality.

It can be seen from the above that assessment of the patient, once they are back in the community, is very important, particularly in psychological terms. Talking through body image problems, relationship problems and problems of complying with treatment regimens can aid a patient's recovery and adaptation, for example:

Mr Jones: I'm glad you've come round, nurse. Seems a long time since I've seen anybody.

Nurse: You sound a bit cross, Mr Jones.

Mr Jones: Well, I can't talk to anybody here.

Nurse: What do you want to talk about particularly?

Mr Jones: Well, it's her, the wife. She hasn't seen the colostomy yet and I don't think she wants to, so like I'm in the spare room.

Nurse: And you don't like that?

Mr Jones: No, but I don't know where to start.

In the above sequence, the nurse discovered that Mr Jones had severe psychological problems with his stoma. He had not accepted it himself, he could not bring himself to show it to his wife but his wife was giving him space and waiting for him to be ready. By talking through the problems with both Mr Jones and his wife separately, the nurse was able to help them to have a conversation together, where, happily, Mrs Jones was quite prepared to accept her husband with his colostomy.

In communicating with patients in this way, there are not always happy endings. Many patients do not adapt readily to the changes brought about by their cancer and some may need referring on through the GP for more expert help. Only through assessment can problems be correctly identified and appropriate action taken.

Towards solutions

The difficulties of adapting to a diagnosis of cancer, once identified, should be put into some order of priority. Many health professionals want to rush in and offer advice for any problem that is identified. The reality is that we can only find solutions to our own problems and this is true for almost every individual. The health professional, when helping patients to adapt to life at home with cancer, should encourage them to identify their own methods of coping. It may be that the patient will identify a problem and the nurse will then ask what they think would help them. The answer may be quite different from what the nurse had expected, or indeed what she would have advised, but it is a fact that the solution identified by the patient may be the one that would work. Only when the patient has exhausted all possibilities in terms of their ideas for solutions to problems should the nurse, doctor or other health professional offer alternatives.

It is often quite hard for health professionals to resist giving advice, particularly if they work in a specialist area. It is well documented, for example, that following mastectomy there is a 25% possibility that the patient will suffer from clinical anxiety or depression, from body image problems and from relationship problems. It is too easy, with this knowledge, to assume that these will be major problems for most mastectomy patients and also that solutions that have worked for other patients may work for this particular patient.

A classic example of giving inappropriate advice came with a woman who had had treatment for cancer of the cervix. She was loath to resume her sexual relationship with her partner because she had read in a women's magazine that cancer of the cervix was either caused by promiscuity or by a partner who was not fussy in the hygiene of keeping his penis and foreskin clean. The patient did not know how to tell her husband how she felt, and the nurse gave advice rather than saying 'What do you think might work?'. The advice given was that the patient should set up a cosy dinner for two and buy steak, red wine and light a candle. The patient listened to the nurse's advice, looking quite surprised, and then said: 'But Jack would think I'm crazy. His favourite food is fish and chips and a glass of Guinness'. What the nurse had not assessed was how this lady dealt with problems in other spheres of her life and what sort of solutions might have worked for her.

Information

In attempting to adapt to life at home with cancer, patients may well need more information than they asked for while they were in hospital. Often they start to think about the future and whether indeed they will have a future. Questions on the disease itself, on current treatment and on the prognosis should be answered as honestly as possible and referred to other sources if the health professional does not have clear answers.

It is important to check what the question means and why it is being asked at a particular time. The classic question 'How long have I got?' is usually asked by individuals who are assessing their own situation and coming to the conclusion that they are perhaps not going to survive their present illness. The acknowledgement of this makes the interaction more comfortable for both parties, as shown in the following exchange:

Mr Beauchamp: Well, how long do you think I've got?

Nurse: I wonder why you're asking me that now?

Mr Beauchamp: Well, I've been thinking. They've sent me home now and told me there's not going to be any more of that terrible treatment, and to tell the truth I'm relieved about that, but I'm not getting better, am I? My weight's going down, I'm not feeling well, I'm always tired and you know I can almost tell from people who visit me – they're not cheerful like they used to be, and my daughter – well, she's got such a worried look and yet when I ask her about it, she says 'No, no'. Either she's got a headache or the wind outside has made her eyes water. They must all think I'm daft.

Nurse: And what are you thinking?

Mr Beauchamp: I'm thinking it won't be long now.

Nurse: Well, I think you're right. I wonder how you feel – bringing that up?

Mr Beauchamp: I guess I'd reached the stage when I needed someone to say 'Yeah, you're getting it right'.

This ability to identify a patient's readiness to talk about the future can be very helpful to the patient, although at the time of the interaction s/he may show signs of being very upset. It is important to give the individual the chance to pick up the pieces and to talk through any worries resulting from having these worst fears confirmed. By sensitive reaction to patients' questions, it is less likely that unwelcome information will be given.

Needs of informal carers

A patient is seldom at home in isolation from other family members. Having the patient discharged into the home when s/he is still needing care can be quite a burden on the relatives. The burden is intensified if the relationship is close and the patient's outlook is poor. There are also problems if the carer is acting from a sense of duty rather than love.

The relative may wish to be present when the health professional sees the patient. In reality, their presence could inhibit the patient from disclosing true concerns. A better arrangement is for the health professional to negotiate with the relative that s/he will get time after the patient has been seen, and this time can be spent in identifying any particular problems. These may be in coping and making arrangements, where appropriate, for help to be made available. There may also be emotional problems that need to be shared, and specific questions and needs for information. Information regarding the patient's disease and outlook should be given with the consent of the patient unless the patient is too ill to be involved with decision-making.

In assessing the needs of carers it sometimes becomes apparent that the patient, being at home, is putting too great a burden on those who care for him. In this situation it may be that the most helpful action for both the patient and his relative is to recommend, through the general practitioner, day care or respite care at the local hospice.

The relatives may need to talk through their guilt if they feel they are not coping, but many will accept some space in order to restore their strength, to take the patient home again, so that their care can continue as before. Relatives may need the opportunity to disclose how tired they are and sometimes to disclose how difficult they find the relative. The charming patient in hospital who endeared themselves to all members of staff may be a very difficult family member at home, particularly when they feel that others have taken over their control of the current situation.

Contracting

Both patients and those who care for them can become very dependent on health professionals who come to their home offering aftercare. Very often the visiting health professional may be the only person who allows the patient and family to talk through their worries and concerns. This means that the visits can be looked forward to and expected to happen more often than is possible.

To avoid dependency relationships, the health professional who is offering aftercare has to make clear ground rules and contracts with the patient and family. At the end of the first visit, which should be about assessment, the health professional will be able to make a decision with the patient and family on how often and for how long the visits should continue.

A Macmillan nurse, for example, might say to a patient: 'I can see that you are settling down quite well at home, but you obviously do have quite a few fears and worries, and I wonder if it would help if I came back and explored some of these further with you?' This allows the patient to say whether they think further visits would be useful and it allows the Macmillan nurse to contract a review date over future visits. In this way, the nurse is giving the patient a clear message: 'You may not always need me'. The terminally ill patient, however, may need regular visits throughout, or may need referring to other agencies.

By contracting in this way, the nurse is encouraging the family to work together with a certain amount of help from outside. This is more healthy for family relationships than if overdependency occurs on one health professional, who is seen as 'the only person who can be of any use to me at this particular time of my life'.

Secondary gains

In communicating with patients in the community who have cancer and who are adapting to a very different life, in terms of both possibilities and length of future, it is usual to expect problems to be concerned with those issues. Many patients, for example, are worried about how much time they have got, what sort of life they are going to have in the time that is available to them, and whether major aims and goals in life are going to be fulfilled.

Emotions may include anger at the current situation, guilt where cancer is seen as a punishment, or blame where it is believed that the current situation could have been avoided if someone had behaved differently. What is not generally expected is that the cancer could have any positive effects on the individual who suffers from it.

Many patients appear to gain some sort of reward for having cancer and when these patients begin to recover, they may feel a sense of loss. For example, Mrs Mathers had cancer of the breast which was followed by a mastectomy and chemotherapy. She made a good recovery and had a reasonably good outlook. She was referred for help by a very confused nurse who could not understand why this patient was not coping with her current situation, given that the outlook was so positive. The reality was that Mrs Mathers lived on her own following a rather messy divorce. Her mother lived round the corner but they had a very ambivalent relationship with much criticism and carping from mother to daughter. Mrs Mathers worked in an office where she was reasonably unhappy and did not have very good relationships with colleagues.

When Mrs Mathers was diagnosed with cancer, her whole life changed. While she was in hospital her mother was transformed in her caring attitude towards her daughter. Colleagues from work brought flowers and fruit and visited regularly in a cheering and caring way. She even had a card from her ex-husband expressing his sorrow that she had such a serious illness.

Mrs Mathers had never previously received such intense loving concern from those people in her life. As she recovered, the situation began to return to normal. Her colleagues, once she was back at work, treated her as they always had, her mother started being difficult again and there was no word from other people in her life. She missed her cancer.

This notion of secondary gains is not well documented but it is something to look out for when identifying problems of cancer patients. Special help may be required to assist the individual to have a more positive outlook on life and to work towards the goal of a better relationship with others that does not depend on need and sympathy.

The cost of effective communication

Whether in hospital or in the community, those who communicate effectively with patients and their families will become much closer to their patient's pain. They will need to look at their own strengths and resources so that they do not take on more work and concerns of other people than they can safely manage. There is a classic syndrome labelled 'burnout', the concept of which comes from America, and which describes the cost of over-involvement in work that is mentally draining. Burnout can be avoided by having a balance between working with patients who are not going to survive and have many problems and those who have a much better outlook. This may mean learning to say 'no' occasionally when asked to see yet another distressed patient, but if health professionals work together as a team it is possible to bring this balance into play so that patients' needs to disclose and discuss their problems are met without one or two professionals taking the major burden.

Clear distinctions need to be made between work and outside life, and certain measures can help this transition to be very clearly identified. For example, those who interact with patients in the community should never give their home telephone number because, once they have, their privacy is invaded. It is much better to give the health centre or hospital telephone number where one can be contacted, in clearly defined time-spans, except in times of emergency.

Many health professionals would describe this protection of self as selfish, but this attitude represents only a short-term view of caring for cancer patients. If the health professional can recognize the cost of working closely with cancer patients and make space for themselves, their friends and their families, they will continue to be able to do the work for a very much longer period than those who give everything and burn out.

References

1   Maguire P and Rutter E (1976) History taking for medical students. Deficiencies in performance. *Lancet* **ii**: 556–8.

2   Faulkner A (1980) *The Student Nurse's Role in Giving Information to Patients*. Steinberg Collection, RCN, London.

3   Maguire P and Faulkner A (1988) How to do it. Improve the counselling skills of doctors and nurses in cancer care. *BMJ*. **297**: 847–9.

4   Fallowfield L and Roberts R (1992) Cancer counselling in the United Kingdom. *Psychology and Health* **6**: 107–17.

5   Faulkner A and Maguire P (1994) *Talking to Cancer Patients and Their Relatives*. Oxford Medical Publications, Oxford.

Further reading

Faulkner A (1992) *Effective Interaction with Patients*. Churchill Livingstone, Edinburgh.

12

Needs assessment in cancer care

D Clark and H Malson

Introduction

Health care reform is now sweeping through many of the affluent nations and is producing new approaches to the development and delivery of services. Everywhere there are concerns about cost containment, efficiency and effectiveness. Long-established assumptions about how and by whom health care should be practised are increasingly subject to new approaches based on regulated markets and managed competition between providers. Whilst new health technologies continue to proliferate, there is a growing determination to subject these to rigorous assessment before they are widely adopted and disseminated and before significant costs are incurred. Within this financially driven set of concerns, some glimmers of true 'reform' are nevertheless in evidence. One of these is the subject of this chapter, in which we shall look at the developing science of health needs assessment as it relates to cancer care. We begin by outlining the key principles of health needs assessment, before moving to an exploration of their application in cancer care. The chapter concludes with an outline of the key benefits that a cancer care needs assessment can offer to cancer care.

Assessing needs: the key principles

In the UK, health commissions or purchasing authorities are responsible for ensuring a comprehensive and integrated range of services for people with cancer, taking into account also the needs of their informal carers. Increasingly, purchasing decisions should be based on systematic assessments of need in local communities with services designed to meet these, emphasizing flexibility and choice. In practice, the process of purchasing cancer services which are 'needs led' is still in its infancy. Relatively little specialist guidance is currently available on the process and implementation in different areas is poorly documented. The task of needs assessment entails reviewing and defining the aggregate needs of a local area based on three dimensions:

- quantitative data (population-based, epidemiological and demographic)

- qualitative data (perspectives of service users, providers, and other key stake-holders)

- comparative data (across different types of service, in different districts and regions and taking into account any national research findings).

The effectiveness of such an assessment depends upon how needs are defined and the ways in which they are measured. There are of course a number of conceptual difficulties surrounding the definition of need, which focus on how broadly need should be perceived for policy purposes. In the context of purchasing for health or social care, need is defined narrowly as the population's ability to benefit from specific services relating to specific problems.[1,2] This definition has two key dimensions. Need is inextricably linked first with service provision, and secondly with the ability to *benefit* from health or social care. It has been pointed out, however, that need does not necessarily equate with demand, which may simply reflect historical circumstances or the interests of particular local clinicians.[3] Similarly supply may not be well matched to need. Within this functional conception of need the ability of the population to benefit from an intervention depends on two things: the incidence and prevalence of a particular condition and the effectiveness of the services available to deal with it. The definition thus embodies a focus on the outcomes of care interventions: if purchasing authorities are to improve health and social well-being, then their aim must be to secure proven, effective provision. The benefit must also be produced at reasonable risk and acceptable cost if it is to be regarded as appropriate for making changes in provision. In a policy context, then, needs are increasingly couched in the language of priorities, addressing questions such as who is to have first claim on limited resources, and who is to judge that claim. In other words, needs are relative, and often have to be traded off against each other, given limited resources.[4]

An important starting point for a cancer-care needs assessment, particularly in the context of supportive care, is the recognition that improvements in well-being and quality of life for people with life-threatening diseases are worthwhile and achievable objectives. Since *palliative* care aims to improve and maintain the quality of remaining life, rather than to cure or prolong life, these considerations should also be taken into account when attempting to assess need. We return to this relatively neglected area in more detail in the following section.

Key dimensions of cancer care needs assessment

Social–epidemiological factors

Epidemiological and demographic data form a major dimension of any assessment of health need. The social and demographic characteristics of a local population, as well as data on the incidence and prevalence of cancer, must inform the planning of services.[5]

Of particular relevance here is the increasing proportion of older people in the population and the increase in diagnoses of cancers. In fact both the incidence and prevalence of most cancers have risen over the last few decades and are expected to continue rising into the next century.[6,7] In 1976 only 2.8 million (4.9% of the total population in England and Wales) were aged 75 or over. By 1984, however, this figure had risen to 3.6 million (6.4%), and it is projected to reach 4.5 million (7.5%) by 2006.[8]

This increase in the number of older people is very relevant to the planning of cancer care services. First because it is associated with the increase in diagnoses of cancers.[9] Older people experience the major impact of cancer.[7,10] In 1988 in England and Wales 65.38% of newly diagnosed cancers and 72.39% of deaths from cancers occurred in those aged 65 and over.[11] With an increase in the number of older people there is, therefore, likely to be a need to expand cancer care services. Second, because the majority of cancers occur in older people, cancer care needs assessments should evaluate the particular psychosocial needs of older people with cancer and the needs of their informal carers, who are themselves also likely to be older.[10,12]

The cancer care needs of a local population will reflect its socio-economic, cultural and ethnic profile as well as its age distribution. The incidence and mortality rates for different forms of cancer have been found to vary between different socio-economic and ethnic groups.[13] For instance, black women have a lower incidence of breast cancer than white women and mortality from smoking-related diseases (including cancers) is significantly associated with increased social deprivation.[14,15] Hence, regional variations in ethnic and socio-economic profiles will be reflected in the local incidence and prevalence of different forms of cancer and hence in the volumes and types of cancer care services that a local population requires. As with age, these factors will also affect the psychosocial needs of people with cancer and their informal carers.

Likewise, the incidence of different forms of cancer vary for men and women. For instance, lung cancer, which accounts for 16% of all new cases, is more than twice as common in men then in women, whilst breast cancer, which accounts for 19% of new cases in women, is rare in men.[9] Women and men will, therefore, have different cancer care needs both because different forms of cancer will require different medical interventions and because they may experience different gender-specific psychosocial needs.

In short, factors such as age, ethnicity and gender, as well as the cultural and socio-economic profile of a population, will determine the prevalence and incidence both of cancers as a whole and of different forms of cancer. They will be reflected in a population's cancer care needs:

- in the volumes of cancer care services required

- in the specific needs of those with different forms of cancer, and

- in the specific psychosocial needs of women and men and of people of different ages and of different ethnic, cultural and socio-economic groupings.

Psychosocial needs

As we have seen, one of the key principles of needs assessment is a commitment to listening to the users of cancer services: taking into account their expressions of need and attending to the psychosocial as well as the medical needs of patients and their informal carers. Indeed, in the UK consultation with users and local people is a central tenet of government legislation in its aim to encourage needs-led (rather than demand- or supply-led) health care service provision.[5,16,17] This is particularly important in the assessment of cancer care needs where, as we noted above, *palliative* care aims to improve and maintain the quality of remaining life, rather than to cure or prolong life. The concept of 'total care', promoted by the hospice movement and others, also stresses the need for psychological, social and spiritual care and for support for informal carers both during a patient's illness and in bereavement.

Recent sociological work on cancer suggests that people with cancer will have particular need of psychosocial support because of social and individual attitudes towards their disease.[18,19] Cancer is often considered to be agonizing, humiliating and inevitably fatal, representing a 'spectacularly wretched' death.[18] People with cancer may also be considered culpable for their own illness because of assumptions that they have an 'unhealthy lifestyle', or that cancer occurs in people of a particular 'emotional type'.[12] Such cultural myths about cancer can only add to a person's difficulties in coping with the illness.

Those with a terminal illness are also likely to need support in coping with the prospect of their own death. Such a task may be particularly difficult in a contemporary Western context in which death is increasingly individualized. Diminishing collective (religious) rites of mourning and the contemporary shift towards informality have left people uncertain about what to do when faced with death.[20] Social fears and vulnerabilities around death may also leave dying people socially unsupported, isolated and even shunned. Elias, for example, has written of the loneliness of many dying people, a loneliness represented in their removal to a hospital and by the increasing withdrawal of others from them.[21] As Elias noted, we often have 'an inability to give dying people the help and affection they are most in need of when parting from other human beings, just because another's death is a reminder of one's own'.[21] In short, social myths and taboos around both cancer and death will increase the difficulties of people with cancer. This need for social and psychological support has been identified in recent cancer care needs assessments. Clark *et al.*, for example, found an expressed need for the company and the social and psychological support that attendance at a day care unit provided.[22] In another study many of the patients and carers similarly expressed the need for counselling as well as home support and respite care.[23] Indeed, there is growing evidence that chronic illnesses such as cancer are associated with psychological distress and that psychosocial interventions are, in general, effective in relieving such distress.[24] Such interventions will not only help patients in adjusting to their illness, reducing depression and anxiety; in some cases they may also extend survival time and reduce costs.[25] Spiegel *et al.* found that women with breast cancer who participated in group therapy lived an average of 18 months longer than women in a control sample, whilst other studies indicate that psychotherapy can result in a 10%–33% reduction in the use of medical services.[27]

As with other areas of health needs assessments, it is also important to assess the particular requirements of different, cultural, ethnic and socio-economic groups, different age groups and the different psychosocial needs of women and men. Such needs may be unmet and poorly understood. Yet in providing cancer care for the whole community it is necessary to understand the cultural and religious belief systems and the particular needs of all its members.

In a multicultural community it will be necessary to provide interpreters and to translate cancer care information into a number of languages. Clark *et al.* found that the 'provision of information appropriately tailored for ethnic minorities and in the community languages continues to be a problem'.[22] There may also be a need for different forms of services that reflect people's different cultural beliefs around health, health care and dying. Such needs can be identified through consultation with service users and the local population, as well as with health care professionals, using qualitative as well as quantitative research procedures.

Similarly, people of different socio-economic backgrounds may hold different beliefs and values around health and health care.[13] Socio-economic factors will also affect health, increased social deprivation being significantly associated with earlier mortality.[13,28] Such structural inequalities have the potential to limit people's health care choices. For example, it is estimated that 56%–58% of cancer patients would prefer to die at home. Yet far fewer achieve this aim, and research suggests that social deprivation is one factor preventing this being achieved.[29] Hence cancer care needs assessments should identify the particular needs associated with social deprivation, enabling appropriate resources to be targeted in a way that acknowledges the impact of social inequalities on cancer care needs. The provision of information not only about diagnosis, prognosis and treatment options but also about available support services and benefits is particularly relevant here.

Men and women can also experience different psychosocial needs because of differences in their expected roles and because their illness may affect their sense of self and their sexuality differently. With the current emphasis on physical appearance women with breast cancer, for example, may need gender-sensitive support in dealing with their illness and their treatment options. Lorde, for example, has written about the guilt that many women with breast cancer experience and psychosocial interventions may be very effective in alleviating such distress.[30]

It is also important to assess access to health education and early detection programmes. It is estimated that 30% of cancer deaths are attributable to tobacco use and 35% to diet.[31] Early detection of malignancies through screening significantly improves prognosis in many cases.[12] Improving access to health care information and screening and identifying areas of unmet needs will therefore have a significant impact on a population's health and on health care costs. Research in the USA has found that black Americans tend to be diagnosed later than their white counterparts and to have poorer outcomes.[32,14] It is possible that such disparities in access to cancer care services also occur in Britain. Older people too may be inadequately screened for a number of reasons.[12] Given the increasing incidence of cancers in older people, it is particularly important that they are targeted with education to promote prevention and early detection.[12] Older people may also have less access to information about their diagnosis because of 'ageist' assumptions that they are unable to cope. Yet in reality many older people will experience less morbidity and depression when they feel they have some choices in life.[12]

In short, the psychosocial aspects of a population's cancer care needs will be many and various. The assessment of cancer care needs must address the particular psychosocial needs associated with cancer and with terminal illness, assessing the needs of potentially isolated and/or distressed patients and carers. In providing for such need it may also be necessary to address the needs of health care professionals. Clark *et al.*, for example, found that many GPs and district nurses felt that training in counselling skills would improve the palliative care services they offered.[22] The assessment of cancer care needs must also address the diversity of psychosocial needs of people of different ages, gender, and ethnic and socio-economic backgrounds. Cancer care needs assessment should identify areas of unmet need in the provision of services and information. It should examine access to services, to information about diagnosis and treatment options and about available services and benefits. It should also examine the cultural sensitivity and accessibility of health care information and screening programmes. Again, it is also important to assess the training needs of health care professionals to enable them to meet the needs of all the members of their community.

Informal carers

It is now well established that appropriate cancer care does not begin and end with the patient. In palliative care especially there is a strong emphasis upon the role of 'informal carers', who may include relatives, neighbours and friends of the sick person. To be comprehensive, any assessment of palliative care needs must therefore include the dimension of informal care.

Whereas it is common for health care providers to talk of the 'primary' and 'secondary' care services, from the perspective of service users both of these are usually seen as supplementary to the provision of self-care and informal care. This is now being recognized by policy-makers, for whom 'care in the community' is increasingly coming to mean care *by* the community. As Neale pointed out, the use of the term 'informal carer' implies a homogeneous group, yet a range of personal and demographic factors will shape and determine the circumstances of individual carers (gender, age, ethnicity, relationship to the cared-for person, and so on).[33] One of the particular features of informal care, as many feminist writers have pointed out, is that it combines labour *and* love and is often motivated by a sense of duty and obligation.[34]

Informal carers of people with cancer may therefore have a wide range of needs, including many of the psychosocial needs discussed in the previous section. Many informal carers are themselves elderly, with health problems of their own. It is important that these are properly recognized in the process of needs assessment and that carers' needs are not inappropriately overshadowed by those of the patient. Carers' own needs and experiences in the context of palliative care have been identified successfully using both survey techniques and qualitative methods.[35,36] Data may be collected retrospectively from bereaved carers or on a prospective basis from those currently caring for someone with a terminal illness. Informal carers are likely to have any combination of the following needs:

- practical support: help with cleaning, cooking, and shopping may be vital when carers feel their sense of movement is restricted by the caring role

- technical information and advice. Several studies have identified the need for clear information and advice on technical and clinical issues, such as lifting and handling, symptom control and pain relief.[22,36] There is a great deal here that health professionals can share which may ease the task of the informal carer. Advice on benefits and financial matters also comes into this category

- emotional support, which may range simply from befriending and providing a 'listening ear', to the full provision of specialist psychological care

- respite care. Caring can be a physically exhausting task, so the provision of respite care is an important service to both the patient and the informal carer. Respite care may take the form of day care or inpatient care. It is not necessarily the domain of highly specialized cancer services and in the UK context, for example, is frequently undertaken by community-based charitable organizations.[37] In the context of protracted periods of informal care, respite provision may prove crucial in enabling the patient to stay at home in the end stages of disease.

Conclusions

What then can health needs assessment offer to cancer care? A number of key benefits can be identified.

There should be a commitment to listening to the users of cancer services (patients and their informal carers), taking into account their expressions of needs. This might include problems and difficulties encountered with particular services or health professionals, as well as identifying areas of satisfaction and examples of good practice. In particular it should focus on areas of need which are only poorly understood from the perspective of health care providers, as well as areas of unmet need. Methodologies for such work can include individual interviews, focus groups and surveys; additional information may be gleaned from complaints documentation.

Taking account of the views of other local stakeholders in the provision of cancer services is also important. This may mean seeking the views of various local community groups concerned with health care, cancer self-help associations, as well as political, religious and other organizations. One exciting technique which has been developed to support this work is that of 'rapid appraisal', whereby health-service managers are required to become researchers for a short period of time in a particular area, meeting local people and forming an assessment of their concerns and how they might be dealt with.[38]

Knowledge gained from these sources can then be set against the views and experiences of health care providers themselves. In this way a more comprehensive picture of 'needs' can be developed and one which is less likely to be dominated by any particular sectional interest. Again, this can be achieved through focus groups, interviews and surveys, as well as modified forms of the Delphi technique.

A thorough understanding of local epidemiological and demographic factors must then be matched to these more qualitative data. This should incorporate an analysis of gender, class and ethnic differences and should take into account locally available data on structured inequalities in health which relate to poverty, housing and employment. Modelling and simulation techniques may be appropriate here in assessing longer-term needs in relation to changing epidemiological and population factors.

As demands grow for health care provision which is both effective and efficient, and as planners strive to tailor provision to the individual circumstances of service users, so the process of needs assessment has come to the fore. We have tried to show here the importance of needs assessment to the continuing development of cancer services, drawing on a variety of perspectives and highlighting a number of appropriate methodologies. In the future comprehensive needs assessment, along the lines we have described, should become the essential prerequisite to service innovation.

References

1 National Health Service Management Executive (1991) *Moving Forward: Needs, Services and Contracts.* NHSME, London.

2 National Health Service Management Executive (1991) *Assessing Health Care Needs: A DHA Project Discussion Paper.* NHSME, London.

3 Stevens A and Gabbay J (1991) Needs assessment needs assessment. *Health Trends.* **23**: 20–3.

4 Williams A (1992) Priorities – not needs. In *Meeting Needs* (eds A Corden, G Robertson and K Tolley), Gower, Avebury, Aldershot.

5 Neale B, Clark D and Heather H (1993) *Purchasing Palliative care: A Review of the Policy and Research Literature.* Occasional Paper 11, Trent Palliative Care Centre, Sheffield.

6 Clegg D (this volume).

7 Lopez A D (1990) Competing causes of death. A review of recent trends in mortality in industrialized countries with specific reference to cancer. *Ann NY Acad Sci.* **609**: 58–74.

8 Central Statistics Office (1987) *Social Trends.* **17**. HMSO, London.

9 Cancer Research Campaign (1989) *Factsheet 1.1 Incidence – UK.*

10 Yancik R and Ries L A (1994) Cancer in older persons: Magnitude of the problem – how do we apply what we know? *Cancer* (Suppl.). **74** (7): 1995–2003.

11 Office of Population Censuses and Surveys (1990) *Cancer Statistics Registration 1985. Series MB1 No. 18 England and Wales.* HMSO, London.

12 Berkman B, Rohan B and Sampson S (1994) Myths and biases related to cancer in the elderly. *Cancer* (Suppl.). **74** (4): 2004–8.

13 Black D (1982) *Inequalities in Health: The Black Report.* Penguin, London.

14 Robertson N L (1994) Breast cancer screening in older black women. *Cancer* (Suppl.). **74** (7): 2034–40.

15 Eames M, Ben-Shlomo Y and Marmot M G (1993) Social deprivation and premature mortality: Regional comparison across England. *BMJ.* **307**: 1097–102.

16   National Health Service Management Executive (1992) *Local Voices: the views of local people in purchasing for health.* NHSME, Leeds.

17   Department of Health (1990) *Contracts for Health Services: Operating contracts.* HMSO, London.

18   Sontag S (1979) *Illness as Metaphor.* Penguin, London, p. 17.

19   Costain Schou K (1993) Awareness context and the construction of dying in the cancer treatment setting: 'micro' and 'macro' levels in narrative analysis. In *The Sociology of Death* (ed. D Clark), Blackwell, Oxford.

20   Mellor P and Shilling C (1993) Modernity, self-identity and the sequestration of death. *Sociology.* **27** (3): 411–37.

21   Elias N (1985) *The Loneliness of the Dying.* Basil Blackwell, Oxford.

22   Clark D, Heslop J and Malson H with Craig B (1995) *'As Much Help as Possible': Assessing Palliative Care Needs in Southern Derbyshire.* Trent Palliative Care Centre, Sheffield.

23   Jones A, Faulkner A and Nightingale S A (1994) *Who cares? Palliative Care Review for United Health Commission (Grimsby and Scunthorpe Health Authority).* Occasional Paper 15, Trent Palliative Care Centre, Sheffield.

24   Hill D R, Kelleher K and Shumaker S A (1992) Psychosocial interventions in adult patients with coronary heart disease and cancer. A literature review. *General Hospital Psychiatry.* **114** (6 Suppl.): 28s–42s.

25   Spiegel D (1994) Health care: Psychosocial support for patients with cancer. *Cancer* (Suppl.). **74** (4): 1453–7.

26   Spiegel D, Bloom J, Kraemer H C *et al.* (1989) Effects of psychosocial treatment on survival amongst patients with metastatic breast cancer. *Lancet.* **2**: 888–92.

27   Mumford E, Schkesinger H J, Glass G V *et al.* (1984) A new look at evidence about reduced cost of medical utilization following mental health treatment. *American Journal of Psychiatry.* **141**: 1145–58.

28   Marmot M G and McDowall M E (1986) Mortality decline and widening social inequalities. *Lancet.* **ii**: 274–7.

29   Higginson I, Webb D and Lessof L (1994) Reducing hospital beds for patients with advanced cancer. *Lancet.* **344**: 409.

30 Lorde A (1980) *The Cancer Journals.* Sheba Feminist Publishers, San Francisco.

31 Doll R and Peto R (1983) *The Causes of Cancer.* Oxford University Press, Oxford.

32 Hardy R and Hargreaves M (1991) Cancer prognosis in black Americans: A mini-review. *Journal of the National Medical Association.* **83** (7): 574–9.

33 Neale B (1991) *Informal Palliative Care: A review of research on needs, standards and service evaluation.* Occasional Paper 3, Trent Palliative Care Centre, Sheffield.

34 Finch J and Groves D (1983) *A Labour of Love: Women, work and caring.* Routledge, London.

35 Seale C and Cartwright A (1994) *The Year Before Death.* Avebury, Aldershot.

36 Neale B (1993) *Informal Palliative Care in Newark: Needs and services.* Occasional Paper 9, Trent Palliative Care Centre, Sheffield.

37 Johnson I, Cockburn M and Pegler J (1988) The Marie Curie/St Luke's relative support scheme: a home care service for relatives of the terminally ill. *Journal of Advanced Nursing.* **13**: 565–70.

38 Cresswell T (1992) Assessing community health and social needs in North Derbyshire using participatory rapid appraisal. *Community Health Action.* **24**, Summer: 12–17.

13

Economics of cancer care

R Akehurst and S Dixon

Introduction

This chapter explains the rationale for undertaking economic evaluations of patient care, and shows that it is not motivated by an obsessive desire to cut costs but by a will to allocate the available budget so as to achieve maximum therapeutic effect. It goes on to discuss and explain the principles and methods of economic evaluation with reference to an illustrative study. A review of how economic evaluation has been used in the past shows that much progress remains to be made in both the quantity and quality of evaluation. The chapter concludes with a discussion of what can be done even when perfect information is not available or an ideal evaluation cannot be undertaken. The relevance of this situation to cancer care in the community is highlighted.

The fundamental economic problem in health care is that the 'capacity to benefit' of the population is so large that not all potentially beneficial treatments can be provided. Even in the wealthiest societies in the world, demands for care run ahead of resources. Health-care resources (e.g. doctors, nurses, equipment and buildings) will always be scarce relative to need, and some services will not be funded. Rationing of services is therefore inevitable and an everyday occurrence in all health-care systems throughout the world. Only the methods of rationing differ.

Economists argue that rationing should further the objective of maximizing the health of the population subject to the overall budget constraint imposed by government. This 'health maximization' can only be achieved by allocating money to those services which represent good 'value for money' ahead of those representing poor value for money. This decision rule means that some services will not be funded or may be funded at a very low level. If this process is followed correctly, however, any reallocation will not be a naive cost-cutting exercise, but rather an informed attempt to increase the aggregate therapeutic effect of the health-care budget.

In order to allocate resources so that health is maximized, information on the effectiveness and cost of services is required. This information may be produced from a variety of sources, a major one being systematic economic evaluation.

What is an economic evaluation?

Economic evaluations are comparative studies in the same way that clinical trials are comparative studies. Particular interventions are compared with the 'do-nothing' (or placebo) approach, 'standard care' or specific alternatives. What defines an economic evaluation is that it embraces both the outcome aspects of interventions and their resources consequences. Knowing costs and health outcomes from a single intervention with no comparator is not helpful when trying to maximize the health of the population. Even the additional costs and benefits compared to 'no active intervention' cannot be ascertained from such descriptive studies, first because even when no active intervention is undertaken, patients will still consume resources such as GP consultations, domicilliary visits, drugs and hospital stays, and secondly because patients will still survive for a period of time without active treatment. Therefore such studies overestimate both the costs and health outcomes associated with the interventions. In fact, many purported economic evaluations are useless because the comparators are not specified clearly enough.

Some descriptive studies focus on the total burden of disease for a given population in terms of cost, morbidity and mortality, and are quite common in the literature. These 'cost-of-illness' studies may form the core of the needs assessment exercises undertaken by health authorities. At best they demonstrate the size of the problem. They say nothing about the amenability of the situation to change or the costs of achieving any change. They also quantify the benefits of the unattainable, i.e. the reduction in costs, morbidity and mortality that would occur if the disease were eradicated. They may have value but such studies are not economic evaluations.

Drummond *et al.* identified four basic types of health care study, of which only one is a true economic evaluation.[1] These are:

- evaluation of costs *or* outcomes *without* a comparison of alternatives. This would generate either a cost description or an outcome description

- evaluation of costs *or* outcomes *with* a comparison of alternatives. This would produce either a cost analysis or an efficacy evaluation (as with a clinical trial)

- evaluation of costs *and* outcomes *without* a comparison of alternatives. This would produce a cost-outcome description (as with cost-of-illness studies)

- evaluation of costs *and* outcomes *with* a comparison of alternatives.

Only studies in the final category are considered to be true economic evaluations and capable of producing information that can help with health maximization. Both cost and outcome measurement are needed in an economic evaluation, both being equally important. As a matter of course, every economic evaluation needs one or more companion clinical evaluations.

Measures of outcome

As was shown above, health economics concerns itself with more than just costs: measurement of patient outcomes is essential. Indeed, outcome measurement is one of the most rapidly developing fields of medicine, and this is partly due to the recent interest of economists. Just as with the other professionals involved in this boom in outcome measurement, such as psychologists, clinicians and nurses, economists approach the problem from their own professional perspective. Consequently, the following discussion looks at measures of outcome for cancer and their relationship to economic evaluation.

In terms of their relevance to economic evaluation, four ways of measuring outcome can be identified. These are set out in Table 13.1 alongside examples. In cancer trials, natural units are the most common, with the most frequently used being one-, three- and five-year survival rates. These have been criticized as they tell us nothing about the quality of life enjoyed by patients who survive over these periods.

Therefore researchers have constructed scales that help to describe and quantify aspects of a patient's quality of life. The information that is needed to rate patients is gathered either by questionnaire, interview or the judgement of clinicians. Quite literally hundreds of such scales exist throughout medicine, of which dozens have been used in oncology. An example is the Karnofsky Performance Status Scale. This assigns values from 0 to 100 (in steps of 10) to describe various states of functioning, such as 'dead' (rated 0), 'disabled', 'requires special care and assistance', 'one self-help skill is prohibited or signifi-

Type of measure	Examples	Form of economic evaluation	Generalizability of results
Natural units	Survival Disease-free survival Time without symptoms and toxicity	Cost-effectiveness analysis (e.g. cost per life year saved)	In limited circumstances the outcome measures and cost-effectiveness ratios may be compared across disease areas
Quality of life	Karnofsky Performance Status Scale Rotterdam Symptom Checklist EORTC QLQ-C30	Cost-effectiveness analysis (e.g. cost per points gained) frequently used as supplementary information to cost-effectiveness analysis using natural units	In limited circumstances the outcome measures and cost-effectiveness ratios may be compared across disease areas
Utility	Euroqol Rosser matrix	Cost-utility analysis (e.g. cost per quality adjusted life year)	Can be compared across disease areas
Willingness to pay	Money	Cost–benefit analysis	Can be compared across disease areas (and in fact with other areas of public expenditure)

Table 13.1: Classification of outcome measures and their associated forms of economic evaluation

cantly impaired' (rated 40), and 'normal', 'no complaints', 'no evidence of disease or impairment' and 'does all activities as usual' (rated 100). These scales have in turn been criticized by some economists on three grounds:

• Many of the scales do not cover all aspects of quality of life.

• Many of the scales just use notional values to rate the various patient descriptions, and as such the numbers are no more than a short-hand numeric description, ordinal in character.

• Many of the scales, even when they value the patient states 'correctly', produce a profile of several dimensions rather than a single index.

Economists have championed the use of utility scales, which aim to resolve the perceived weaknesses of other scales listed above. The first of these was the Rosser index, which measured quality of life along two dimensions: pain and disability. The matrix produced from these two dimensions assigned values to the various patient states described so that a change from 0.1 to 0.2 was valued by people the same as a change from 0.75 to 0.85. Zero was the value given to death, and unity the value given to perfect health. This has been superseded by the Euroqol, a utility measure that covers six dimensions of quality of life (mobility, self-care, main activities, social relationships, pain and mood).

Another way of measuring the value of a change in health status that is used solely by economists (and even then only very rarely) is a person's willingness to pay for the improvement. This does not mean that patients have to pay for the treatment being researched: money is used only as the gauge of improvement. This enables the benefits of treatment as valued by the patients to be compared directly with the costs of providing the treatment. It is a highly contentious method of valuation.

Guidelines on the use of quality of life measures in cancer patients were issued by the MRC's Cancer Therapy Committee Working Party on Quality of Life in 1989, but they are in desperate need of revision.

Types of economic evaluation

The generalizability of the conclusions that can be drawn from an economic evaluation are related to the type of evaluation undertaken, which in turn is determined by the outcome measures used. This means that when designing a clinical trial/economic evaluation, health professionals and economists need to work closely so that the outcome measures used are both clinically relevant and capable of answering the economic questions of importance. Table 13.1 shows what can be done with the results of each form of economic evaluation.

Cost-effectiveness ratios from one evaluation should only be compared with other such ratios if the dimension of outcome used in the ratio is dominant or if other dimensions of outcome (such as quality of life) are judged to be the same for the treatments. This means that only in very limited circumstances should the results of cost-effectiveness studies in cancer be compared with studies in other disease areas, and secondly that some comparisons within cancer should not be undertaken using cost-effectiveness analysis.

The overall role of quality of life measures in health economics is currently being debated but, in terms of cost-effectiveness analysis, only in very special circumstances can quality of life instruments be used.

The results of cost–utility analysis (e.g. cost per quality-adjusted life year (QALY)) – can be used to compare interventions across all disease areas, such as hip replacements, chemotherapy for small-cell lung cancer (SCLC) and heart transplantation. The implication of this is that it can inform priority-setting exercises not only within cancer services, for instance, but also priority setting between cancer services and other parts of the health service.

Cost–benefit analysis can be used to compare between any interventions, and is the only form of analysis that can indicate quantitatively whether the benefits outweigh the costs. However, its use remains controversial. It was used, albeit very rarely, in the UK in the last decade. It is a more common form of evaluation in the USA and is enjoying something of a renaissance of interest on the European side of the Atlantic.

An example of the potential use of economic evaluation

To demonstrate the potential value of economic evaluation, an example of how one could be used to help resolve uncertainty in a single aspect of cancer treatment is briefly described below. The example is not meant as a comprehensive and definitive description nor as an indication of its importance.

Several clinical evaluations have assessed the benefits of prophylactic cranial irradiation (PCI) in patients with SCLC, and while there is good evidence to show that it reduces the risk of cranial relapse, the effects on survival are ambiguous. If an economic evaluation were to be set up to run alongside a new randomized controlled trial of PCI vs no PCI in SCLC, information additional to baseline clinical measures would need to be gathered. A guide to this information is given in Table 13.2, although the choice of outcome measures may overlap with the clinical information that may be gathered, and there is probably no consensus amongst economists over which measures should be used. (A clinical trial aimed at resolving this problem is currently ongoing and is using the Rotterdam Symptom Checklist and the Hospital Anxiety and Depression Scale as measures of quality of life.)

The information given in Table 13.2, and the subsequent economic evaluation, would add to a 'basic' clinical trial of PCI in patients with SCLC in a number of ways. First, it would allow any differences to be identified on the

Type of data		Items
Cost	Hospital	Equipment costs
		Staff costs
		Inpatient costs
		Outpatient costs
	Primary care	GP contacts
		Drug costs
	Community care	Macmillan nurse costs
		District nurse costs
	Indirect costs	Time off work by patient and carer
Outcomes		Euroqol
		EORTC QLQ-C30

Table 13.2:   Information required for an evaluation of prophylactic cranial irradiation

basis of a single index measure of outcome (e.g. the Euroqol). In conventional trials, information from patient diaries, checklists, survival rates and so on, will only rarely produce an unambiguous answer as one treatment is unlikely to dominate the comparator treatment on all measures of outcome. Utility measures (such as the Euroqol) contain information on many aspects of quality of life that has been aggregated to produce an overall 'answer'.

Secondly, it would measure the difference in cost between the groups. This would measure the cost of PCI and also the resource consequences of the treatment. These consequences could be very important. For example, if the treatment causes any neurofunctional impairment, extra costs of care will be incurred. Alternatively, if the treatment reduces the rate of cranial relapse, these patients may use fewer resources in the future as they will be less incapacitated by the progression of the disease than those who do suffer brain metastases. It should be noted that capturing the full economic effects in an evaluation may involve collecting data to a later endpoint than would be the case if a clinical study alone were being performed.

Finally, it would allow the value for money of the treatment to be calculated using a cost per QALY. If this were high (perhaps due to poor patient response, treatment side effects and large cost consequences), it may be concluded that if no PCI is given to these patients the additional costs could be used to greater therapeutic effect elsewhere for cancer patients. Alternatively, if the cost per QALY were low (due to good patient response in terms of quality of life and lower than expected costs due to small cost consequences of treatment), it may be concluded that money should be freed from elsewhere in the cancer (or general health service) budget to fund the service.

A complete evaluation would undertake marginal analysis to identify whether the cost and outcome relationships were such that the ratio of cost/QALY changed with level of provision. This might make provision a good idea up to a certain level, but not thereafter.

The capability of measuring many different dimensions of patient outcome within a single index and the 'value for money' of the treatment are achieved through the economic evaluation. It is only an economic evaluation that can be used to judge whether the provision of the service is likely to add to or reduce the total amount of health gain produced from a given budget. A complication, of course, is that there may not be one coherent budget but several. For example, some costs may fall on a local authority, some on the NHS and some on individuals. Separate analysis of the different budgets may be needed, or of one, depending on the perspective of the study.

Published economic evaluations

Despite the need for economic evaluations, very few have been undertaken. In fact, even the most basic information on the efficacy of most treatments used in the health service today is lacking. On the back of this, most economic evaluations published in journals are of poor quality. This is due mostly to a lack of understanding of even the most basic standards of good practice by many, and the evolving form of economic evaluation, which is still in its infancy.

The small number of economic evaluations (and their recent growth) can be seen from an analysis of an economic evaluation bibliography published in 1992 by Backhouse *et al.*.[2] Figure 13.1 shows that there has been an almost exponential growth in published economic evaluations of cancer services over the past 25 years.

Only 170 economic evaluations were identified in the bibliography. Many of these are crude cost-of-illness studies, and indeed are not strictly economic evaluations. Furthermore, no evaluations of community cancer services are in this bibliography. The vast majority of research money is allocated to the more glamorous area of hospital medicine. This is beginning to change with a growing recognition by funding bodies of the relative importance of palliative and community care.

With such a small pool of studies, even if one that is of interest were to be found, there is still a profound risk that one of the following would apply:

• It will be of such poor quality that it is of little use.

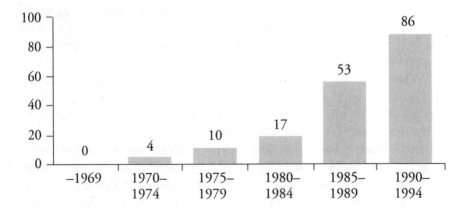

Figure 13.1:   Number of published economic evaluations of cancer services.

• It is good quality but the results are not generalizable to local circumstances (e.g. due to a different case-mix of cancers).

• It is of good quality and generalizable, but the information is not presented in such a way that it can be adapted to your local circumstances (e.g. a different configuration of community services means that the costs used are not applicable).

Only very rarely will the results of a published study be capable of being directly transferable to your local circumstances without further local analysis. The best long-term strategy for tackling these problems is to undertake more good economic evaluations. However in the short term, use can be made of data that are already available in the literature and the health service, through simple modelling techniques such as decision analysis.[3] These techniques are being increasingly used by economists to remedy poor studies, and even to generalize the results of good studies.

The shortage of economic evaluations involving cancer care in the community, as shown in Figure 13.1, means that such modelling techniques could be of great value in evaluating the cost-effectiveness of community cancer care.

Conclusions and way forward

Economic evaluation is a relatively new technique in medicine and it is being increasingly used to provide much-needed information to help with producing the maximum amount of therapeutic effect from the funds available to provide health care. However, the fact that it is in its infancy means that this information is still in short supply. Progress needs to be made, and this is best achieved through:

- developing a better understanding of economic evaluation techniques so that past examples of poor evaluations can be identified (and avoided)

- using past evidence to the best possible effect through the modelling of costs and outcomes

- widespread use of economic evaluation techniques alongside clinical trials.

References

1   Drummond M F, Stoddart G L and Torrance G W (1987) *Methods for the Economic Evaluation of Health Care Programmes.* Oxford University Press, Oxford.

2   Backhouse M E, Backhouse R J and Edey S A (1992) Economic evaluation bibliography. *Health Econ.* **1** (Suppl.): 1–235.

3   Thornton J G, Lilford R J and Johnson N (1992) Decision analysis in medicine. *BMJ.* **304**: 1099–103.

14

Purchasing and providing cancer care

B D Aird and H C Orchard

Introduction

It is a well known fact that one in three people will develop cancer at some time in their life. This represents an enormous volume of work and consumption of resources within all sectors of the NHS. The current pattern of services and the way in which they are purchased have developed in a relatively ad hoc manner, and many health-care professionals recognize the inadequacies in the provision of modern comprehensive care for patients with cancer. However, recent impetus for a radical change in the organization of service delivery has arisen from the Chief Medical Officer. This chapter therefore outlines the current mechanism by which cancer care is purchased and provided in the UK, indicates some of its inherent problems, and looks forward to the future structure and the challenges it presents.

The current purchasing/providing framework

The care and treatment of cancer do not fit easily into the current purchasing and providing framework of the NHS. The complex nature of the disease means that there are a variety of settings in which care can be most appropriately provided at different stages of illness. A patient may receive treatment from a large number of health-care professionals working for various different organizations and at different levels of specialization. At the primary level, care is provided by GPs, district nurses and other specialist nurses. Chest physicians, general surgeons, urologists, gynaecologists and haematologists provide the bulk of secondary care from local district general hospitals. Tertiary services are provided by cancer specialists – clinical oncologists (radiotherapists) and medical oncologists – in specialist oncology units, which may be part of teaching hospitals, or independent NHS trusts. In addition, the high-profile nature of the disease attracts much by way of support from the voluntary and charitable sectors, who form a significant body of small service providers which, to a greater or lesser degree, are privately funded. The potential involvement of so many agencies in the treatment of one patient can lead to fragmentation in the delivery of care and difficulties in maintaining any sense of continuity. There are also disadvantages for the purchaser as specific aspects of care are bought from separate providers, and the overall view of the requirements of groups of patients with a particular disease type can be lost. The current framework and some of its inherent problems are discussed below.

Purchasing cancer care

The purchasing of cancer care is managed through the same mechanism as most other aspects of clinical service in the NHS – the contracting cycle. The cycle begins with the purchaser determining the health-care priorities of its resident population and publishing its intentions in its annual purchasing plan. Currently the only purchasers of tertiary cancer care are district health authorities (DHAs), as GP fundholders do not receive funding to buy these services. They do, however, purchase care within the secondary setting and, with moves in the foreseeable future towards total purchasing for GP fundholders, it is possible that GPs will gain responsibility for purchasing an increasing range of care for patients with cancer. Nevertheless, it is likely that there will always be some aspects of cancer care – the high-cost, low-volume treatments – which are purchased on a district-wide basis.

District health authorities assess their purchasing priorities in conjunction with imperatives that have been determined locally and set nationally. The national imperatives that play a large part in influencing the purchasers' agenda for cancer services are those specified in the *Health of the Nation* document.[1] Cancers were a major area focused on by the *Health of the Nation*, with targets being set for reductions in death rates for breast and lung cancer and the incidence of cervical and skin cancers. The very act of attempting to set targets highlighted the problem of the lack of data on the outcomes of cancer treatment and the difficulties in measuring the effects of treatment interventions. Most purchasers have begun to address the relevant targets in their annual purchasing plans. It is generally the case, however, that although the targets specify that reductions in death rates should be made, as well as halting or reducing incidence, thus far purchasers have generally concentrated their efforts on prevention and screening. Priorities for investment have therefore revolved around health promotion initiatives and screening services rather than on improved treatment options for people who already have cancer.

Local imperatives are determined primarily by the health needs assessment work undertaken by DHA public health clinicians. However, GPs are playing an increasingly important role in influencing the local purchasing strategies of DHAs through various models of primary-care-led purchasing, such as 'locality purchasing' and the more radical 'total fundholding' experiments. Whilst the objective of this work is usually to bring the benefits of fundholding to the whole population, the more immediate practical impacts have included greater innovation in arranging service delivery and a marked willingness to challenge poor provider performance and move contracts elsewhere. Thus if a district discovers that its incidence of a particular type of cancer is above the national average, and consequently chooses to target additional resources into this area, its choice of the provider with whom to place the annual contract will generally have been made on a historical basis. More recently, and largely as a result of GP involvement, purchasers have begun to identify areas in which a shift in the type or location of care for a group of patients is judged to be desirable and to begin the gradual implementation of such policies. One example of this might be a strategy to enable cancer patients in the terminal stages to die at home if they so wish, rather than in a hospital or hospice, and consequently to purchase an increased level of community nursing services. The longer-term implications of the influence of GPs on purchasing are not yet clear but are likely to be far-reaching.

Contracts in their current format tell a purchaser little about what they are actually buying, nor do they give much indication of the quality of care. In particular, treatment provided at secondary level is generally swallowed up within the overall medical and surgical contracts held by the hospital. Contracts with tertiary units provide little more than an indication of the number of patients treated without specifying how they were treated or what they were treated for. Contracting currencies, which may be expressed in finished consultant episodes (FCEs) or bed days, day cases and outpatient attendances, do not reflect the case-mix of the patients. An increase in the number of patients needing complex treatments requiring a high level of technical support or complex chemotherapy regimens, with the consequent resource implications, is therefore not represented in the current contracting framework for cancer services. A serious stumbling block in the development of more effective contracts, however, is the lack of knowledge and understanding on the part of purchasers about oncology treatment. This is partly due to the fact that, until recently, most specialist cancer treatments were purchased on a regional basis and so DHAs did not have to grapple with the problems inherent in oncology services. But it is exacerbated by the speed and range of developments in treatments. Technological advances in radiotherapy and increasingly sophisticated chemotherapy regimens are continually improving the treatment options for patients with cancer. In order for purchasers to increase their effectiveness, a programme of continuing education and updating is therefore necessary.

Providing cancer care

Whilst it is generally the case that the first health professional the cancer patient comes into contact with is the GP, the majority of his or her treatment will take place in secondary and tertiary settings. A significant amount of treatment is provided within district general hospitals by clinicians who are specialists in their own right – such as surgeons and gynaecologists – but are unlikely to have had any formal specialist training in the non-surgical management of cancer. The contribution of these clinicians is primarily surgical, but a substantial amount of chemotherapy is also prescribed in DGHs by doctors who are not cancer specialists, giving rise to some concern about the quality assurance of such treatment. Many DGHs are served by visiting cancer specialists, primarily radiotherapists, who run outpatient clinics to which the DGH's consultants refer new patients and in which follow-up patients can be seen locally.

Tertiary services are provided at centralized oncology centres which, for the most part, offer radiotherapy, medical oncology and sophisticated diagnostic facilities. They may also have available specialist surgical services, bone marrow transplantation and facilities for treating paediatric cancers. At least one tertiary centre exists in each region: centralized planning has played a part in the location of most radiotherapy departments due to the high capital cost of the equipment. Nevertheless, many patients have to travel long distances to centres for radiotherapy treatment on an outpatient basis, and some travel for consultations with a specialist doctor where no outreach arrangements exist.

Where possible, patients return to the community for rehabilitation and palliative and terminal care. It is here that specialist nursing staff, working with the GP and other doctors involved in the patient's care, provide much of the support needed to ensure that treatment programmes are maintained and that the patient does not need readmission to hospital. Patients who cannot be cared for at home may be admitted to a hospice for the purposes of facilitating symptom control or intensive nursing during terminal care.

Without doubt, the current organization of cancer care in the UK contains some areas of excellence, but of primary concern to purchasers and providers alike is that these high standards are not replicated throughout the service. The fragmented way in which services have developed over the last few decades has resulted in inequality of access to timely specialist treatment for some sections of the population. Clearly the number of patients affected by this disease and the associated resource implications demanded a revision of existing systems and the development of a new model to manage the delivery of comprehensive care to cancer patients.

The future purchasing/providing framework

In April 1995, the Expert Advisory Group on Cancer under the leadership of the Chief Medical Officer Dr Kenneth Calman published a report entitled *A Policy Framework for Commissioning Cancer Services.*[2] The purpose of this document was to establish a pattern of purchasing cancer services (and therefore by implication a pattern of service delivery) which ensured that patients with cancer were detected, diagnosed and treated in the most appropriate place and as early as possible.

To achieve this objective, the report proposed that care should be purchased at three levels:

- at the primary care level

- at designated cancer units

- at designated cancer centres.

The primary care level was seen as the focus of care, the expectation being that links between GPs and secondary hospital services would be strengthened and appropriate patterns of referral and follow-up would be established.

Designated cancer units in local hospitals would be of sufficient size to support multidisciplinary clinical teams, with sufficient expertise and facilities to manage the more common cancers. Each cancer unit would require a local coordinator to ensure that services dovetailed and that appropriate levels of expertise were being applied across the service. The coordinator would also be expected to ensure that non-surgical oncology services, mostly provided on a visiting basis, linked with local surgical services. Implications of this model include the need for further subspecialization in surgery (to ensure that any doctor practising cancer surgery undertook a minimum caseload) and the inevitability that not all general hospitals would be capable of becoming cancer units in their own right.

Designated cancer centres would provide an extra range of specialized services at the tertiary level in support of cancer units. They would also treat less common cancers or provide treatments which were too technically demanding, too specialized or too capital intensive for cancer units. These cancer centres would normally serve a population in excess of one million people and would be characterized by a high degree of specialization and comprehensive provision of all the facets of care necessary in modern cancer management.

The report also proposed a further subcategory – a cancer unit with radiotherapy – where, primarily for geographical reasons, it would be necessary to provide radiotherapy services in a cancer unit which is not large enough to support the full range of activity of a cancer centre.

One result of these proposals is an inevitable emphasis on the development of the so-called 'hub-and-spoke' model of provision, where the hub is the cancer centre and the spokes are outreach from the centre to the cancer units. In order to achieve the benefits of a high degree of specialization in addition to local provision this model demands that the cancer centre provides non-surgical oncology expertise in the cancer unit (a minimum of five sessions per week was the recommendation), as well as outreach chemotherapy services. In the opposite direction, one would expect to see the rarer and more complex cancers being referred quickly from the cancer unit to the cancer centre.

It is clear that simply designating cancer units and cancer centres will not in itself achieve the benefits of local provision and high specialization along with appropriate referral. This can only be made possible through the development of clinical guidelines and protocols which describe the clinical relationships between different levels of care and deal with the way in which particular disease sites should be handled in relation to diagnosis, treatment and continuing care. The development of these guidelines must obviously be led by doctors and include primary, secondary and tertiary levels to ensure that the patient's needs are catered for in a seamless and continuous service.

From the purchasing perspective, once these guidelines are established it is possible to begin to think seriously in terms of purchasing 'packages of care' which span the whole spectrum of care, from primary, through secondary to tertiary care and back to the community. This is an attractive proposition to purchasers, who are concerned to ensure that the patient has access to a comprehensive and integrated range of services delivered in the appropriate place and at the appropriate time, having regard to the progress of the patient's disease. It also opens up the possibility, in the longer term, of linking purchasing strategies directly to health outcomes.

From the provider perspective, it opens the door to the creation of highly specialized service providers delivering a range of care through contracts and subcontracts in a variety of locations, freed from the constraints of existing physical or Trust boundaries. This notion of a specialist provider delivering services in a 'shop within a shop' is common enough in the private sector but has yet to make an impact on the NHS.

Challenges ahead for purchasers and providers

It is clear that if purchasers and providers are to succeed in implementing the recommendations of the Expert Advisory Group on Cancer many difficult challenges will need to be tackled over the next few years. Quite apart from the logistics of shifting to this pattern of purchasing and provision, the two biggest implications are likely to be the need for an increased number of specialists to deliver what is essentially a much higher standard of care and treatment, and information provision for contracting.

At the present time, medical manpower plans have not allowed for an increased number of oncology specialists and, given the lead time necessary to create additional doctors, this presents an enormous challenge to the health-care system. The problem of availability of medical staff will be further exacerbated by the mandatory process of reaccreditation for consultants.

Furthermore, information provision for contracting in cancer care is crude and patchy. The development of clinical guidelines and 'packages of care' will only benefit purchasing and provision if it is underpinned by more flexible, more comprehensive and more robust information systems. Purchasers need population data on the expected number of cases, health services data to quantify anticipated activity and workload by specialty and provider, data on evaluations of interventions and services, and the ability to monitor outcomes.

The challenges will not, however, simply be of an organizational or clinical nature. Decisions of an economic and ethical character will be unavoidable if services are to be radically improved. The rise in public awareness about health in general and new treatments in particular (with the subsequent demand for them to be available on the NHS), coupled with the gradual increase in the incidence of cancer in the population, will force purchasers to examine their priorities for resource consumption. A clear commitment to purchase on the basis of need rather than demand is required, but this will be politically and ethically sensitive. The concept of rationing is a particularly difficult one to apply to cancer, which is an 'emergency' specialty with a high proportion of palliative, non-curative work. Providers are, however, already expected to identify areas for 'disinvestment' where specific treatments are not of proven effectiveness, so that purchasers can withdraw funds to reinvest elsewhere in the system. The lack of available data on the quality outcomes of cancer treatment, as well as the close relationship between research and service provision, with clinical trials (by their very nature 'unproven'), playing such an important role, renders this a hazardous undertaking.

The key to achieving success in these areas will lie partly in the availability and use of improved information on the number and type of procedures undertaken and their effectiveness as determined by clinical audit. However, the volume of work to be undertaken to establish robust protocols that are acceptable to clinicians and usable within a purchasing framework is immense and will require further investment and collaborative working between DHAs and all providing sectors. The challenge for all parties will be in keeping pace with the continual evolution and change in the field of cancer treatment even whilst 'packages of care' are being specified, in order that meaningful contracting mechanisms can be developed that reflect what actually happens to the patient and the consequent resource implications. This may result in the establishment of purchasing consortia or 'lead purchaser' arrangements for cancer so that the vast knowledge necessary for effective purchasing is concentrated in specific areas, and the number of parties with whom cancer centres in particular have to contract is reduced.

The programme for change in the organization of cancer care and treatment over the next five years is enormous. It represents a real opportunity for clinicians and managers to improve significantly the quality and accessibility of services for one of the largest groups of patients coming through the doors of the NHS. This opportunity will be missed, however, unless purchasers and providers develop mature relationships between and among themselves, enabling them to work alongside each other to make these changes. A spirit of cooperation and communication will be essential if the necessary networks are to be established and expertise shared among professionals, so that the greatest benefit can be realized for the patient.

Summary

- Cancer care is purchased primarily by DHAs, who assess the needs of their population and then agree contracts with provider units.

- The wide range of providers who have an input into the care of a cancer patient – from primary through to tertiary specialists – makes purchasing services a complex task.

- Contracts for cancer care are in the early stages of development and currently provide little information about treatments used and their outcomes.

- A recent report from the Chief Medical Officer recommended the reorganization of cancer services in Britain to improve access and quality of care for patients.

- Achieving the goals of this report will require closer collaboration between purchasers and providers to tackle the organizational, clinical, economic and ethical challenges ahead.

References

1 Department of Health (1992) *Health of the Nation. CM1986.* HMSO, London.

2 Expert Advisory Group on Cancer (1995) *A Policy Framework for Commissioning Cancer Services.* Department of Health, London.

Index